Path OF
FIRE AND
LIGHT
Advanced Practices of Yoga

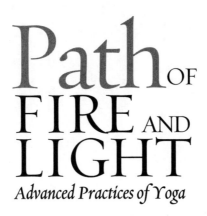

Path OF FIRE AND LIGHT

Advanced Practices of Yoga

Swami Rama

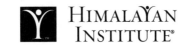

HIMALAYAN INSTITUTE

HONESDALE, PENNSYLVANIA USA

Himalayan Institute
952 Bethany Turnpike
Honesdale, PA 18431

HimalayanInstitute.org

Printed in the United States of America

25 24 23 22 21 20 19 18   7 8 9 10

ISBN-13: 978-0-89389-097-1 (paper)

Library of Congress Cataloging in Publication Data
Rama, Swami

> Path of fire and light.
> Includes index.
> 1. Breathing exercises. 2. Yoga, Hatha. I. Title.

RA782.R34 1986   613.7'046   86-7586

♾ This paper meets the requirements of ANSI/NISO Z39-48-1992
(Permanence of Paper).

CONTENTS

FOREWORD

The highest accomplishments in any art or science are the product of patient effort. A violinist plays the Beethoven concerto or a physician performs an organ transplant only after years of preparation. Without such intense preparation, no art or science can really develop.

Thus it is with yoga. Sleeping skillfully, eating wisely, breathing well—these are the first steps on the path. They are commonplace, but deceptively so. Rather than diminishing in importance, these themes become increasingly significant as practice levels intensify. As you will see, advanced yoga practices challenge imagination and raise everyday life to rarified levels of awareness.

At present, yoga is largely identified with *asana* practice. This means that advanced yoga is often expected to consist simply of advanced postures. But while there is enormous value in working with yoga asanas, that is not the aim of this book. Here you will learn about the highly refined techniques of *pranayama* and meditation, only rarely described with authenticity. Most important, this book tells of self-unfoldment—about the precise ways in which yogis, past and present, have directly approached the transcendent within themselves. This is the highest realm of practice, the final stage of the journey of yoga.

That journey must, of course, begin somewhere. The *Yoga Vasishtha*, an early yogic text, says that there are four gatekeepers at the entrance to the path of self-unfoldment: self-control, contentment, good company, and inquiry into the nature of the Self. Self-control, says the text, is the source of everything good and auspicious. It is the remedy for physical and mental ills, and with it, even food is said to taste better. Contentment is the source of happiness. It is the product of finding fulfillment in what comes unsought.

Good company is said to be superior to every other spiritual observance—better than pilgrimage, charity, and fasting. It means keeping company with those who have realized some measure of truth, whose uncertainty is therefore dispelled, and whose happiness is well established. The spirit of inquiry prompts a person to study scriptures, to ask about the nature of the Self, and to hold to tranquility even in the face of great sorrow. This leads to meditation and to a path of stillness.

Building on these qualities and skillfully merging them with classical yoga practice, this book offers a remarkable vision of yoga. It is based on Sanskrit texts such as the *Yoga Sutra* of Patanjali (c. 1st century BCE) and the *Hatha Yoga Pradipika* of Swatmarama (c. 15th century CE). But it is equally grounded in the experience of its author, an accomplished yogi whose life was shaped through early training with many of the greatest saints and personages of 20th-century India. Raised under the guidance of a brilliant *sadhu* (spiritual ascetic) whose yogic attainment was legendary, Swami Rama received both singular training in the practices of yoga and a modern education in the finest schools and universities of North India. Along the way he became a young acquaintance of Gandhi, a spiritual brother of Tagore, a student of the great Indian philosopher Ranade, and an acclaimed sadhu under his master's guidance.

He came to the United States to teach in the late 1960s during a period in which paradigms of Western medical thought were being transformed. Displaying an astonishing degree of self-mastery in the laboratories of the Menninger Foundation, he showed that control of internal functioning is well within the capacity of human consciousness. His demonstrations were widely known (they were summarized in the 1973 *Encyclopedia Britannica Yearbook of Science*), fueling further research and buoying the newly developing fields of biofeedback and alternative medicines. But Swami Rama never considered his demonstrations to be more than a preliminary indication of the potentials of yoga. Thus, it was that after many years of teaching in the West, years in which he carefully presented the basic elements of yoga to his students, Swami Rama finally chose to speak about advanced practice.

Those who were fortunate enough to learn from him during his lifetime will recognize in this book Swami Rama's characteristic style of writing and speaking. He presented teachings in a manner that carefully respected and preserved the work of the great yogis of the past. But his writing about matters of advanced practice often reflected personal experience. Many students have remarked that because of this, both his word selection and manner of organizing thoughts are uniquely evocative.

In regard to the content of this book, a few reflections may be helpful. Swami Rama writes in chapter five:

> In tantric philosophy, a human being is seen as being like a miniature universe or a microcosm that parallels the whole of the external manifestation, the macrocosmic universe. The principles that govern the universe also govern every individual.

What are those principles, and how do they govern individual life? In a sense, this entire book is an elegant answer to these questions. It begins with the recognition of each individual's relationship to the cycles of day and night, to the nutritional powers of food, and to the breathing patterns that directly link him or her with the universe. Breath, in its highest form, is a manifestation of a universal energy: *shakti*. It flows as living energy: *vayu*. But its flow is resisted by the effects of a false sense of egoism: the accumulation of negative *karma*. A practitioner who recognizes these three great motifs will find in them the organizing principles for every level of experience. In advanced practice, shakti is the inclination toward self-realization; vayu is the medium of motion or "that which flows" (in this book, largely defined as the breath and its subtle operations); and karma is the force of resistance that restrains the impetus toward Self-realization. According to Swami Rama, an advanced yogi seizes the ability to voluntarily control breathing in order to overcome negative karma and reveal the Self.

As fascinating as advanced techniques may be, descriptions about them can feel overwhelming, overly mechanical, or both. Is it really possible, for example, for vast powers of consciousness to be awakened merely by manipulating one's breath? With the restraint characteristic of a careful teacher, Swami Rama subtly discourages students from thinking so. It is not technique alone, but technique augmented with understanding that matters. Thus, in every chapter, the book provides a philosophical context for the practices described there.

Like a piece of music layered with various colors, textures, and moods, you will discover numerous strata in this book. It relates the need for yoga, describes the specific disciplines that bring success in its practice, and clarifies the strategies that can help in removing obstacles along the way. It takes the sting out of many Sanskrit terms, leaving one wanting to learn more about the nuances of this ancient language. It presents a striking vision of life, an explanation in words and symbols that is both practical and transformative. And it awakens the aspiration, as practice evolves, to understand at least some of these disciplines for yourself.

I suspect that you will find *Path of Fire and Light* worth reading more than once. With each reading, new impressions are lodged and new lessons learned. In the end, you may well discover that the practice you are doing has not changed substantially, yet it has matured. Advanced practice, it seems, is your own practice—the practice you do—filled with new understanding.

Rolf Sovik, PsyD
Spiritual Director, Himalayan Institute

INTRODUCTION

The subject matter of this book is the advanced practices of yoga, condensed from ancient scriptures. I have endeavored to verify and examine the authenticity of these exercises myself, and I visited and sat at the feet of those who completely devoted their lives to attaining the goal of life. I was fortunate to meet a few who walked on the path of light, and who denied the existence of darkness by saying that the sun itself never knows what darkness looks like. It is only the ignorant who live in the darkness of ignorance, not the enlightened ones. But who are these enlightened ones?

In all great cultures there have been great people, torchbearers, who, through their wisdom, have helped many on the path of truth. Their existence assures humanity that human beings are able to walk on the path of light if they follow the instructions imparted by the great ones and practice.

Interior research is fundamentally different from the research conducted in the external world. In the external world the researcher finds subjects for his experiments, but in interior research the researcher must become the subject himself. This task is enormously difficult, for the interior researcher must assume the attitude, "I am a researcher, I am a laboratory, and I am the subject." To have the conviction that one can successfully pursue this approach, one must first gather sufficient information by studying the scriptures and visiting those teachers who really practice.

If he is to attain the truth, there must be an unflickering flame burning in the heart of the aspirant. This arises when one has carefully examined the external world and finds that the external world is just a small particle of the vast universe. Anything that occurs in the external world has actually already occurred within long before, though the cause remains hidden. When one awakens to this fact and is fully convinced that life in the external world is not completely satisfying, then he turns within in search of the truth. A true researcher uses all means available to search for the cause of external events in the internal world. He wants to know the truth; he wants to understand life within as well as he understands it outside himself.

The way of knowing the external world is entirely different from the way of knowing the internal states of a human being. In the former, one proceeds from the gross to the grosser and then toward the grossest. The latter is from the gross to the subtle and then to the subtlest. Only a few dare to tread this second path, for it is the path of the unknown. There is a saying that when a student searches, the teacher appears. It is true. It is true that when one sincerely searches for truth with all his mind, action, and speech, he attains it.

The most ancient science is yoga science. It is as ancient as human existence. But, alas, it was practiced by only a fortunate few and has not become a part of the educational system of society. Perhaps modern man does not undertake this research for two reasons. First, the practices of yoga science require that time be set aside, and modern man is caught in the whirlpool of his own creations and expectations which keep him uselessly busy. So there is a cry from seekers: "We don't have enough time." The second problem is fear of the unknown. Those who are awakened have begun to realize that the purpose of life cannot be fulfilled solely by an external way of living. They start organizing their lives and adjust themselves in such a way that they have time to feel the innermost urge to know truth and understand their internal states. Such aspirants start treading the path of light.

To tread the path of inner light one looks here, there, and everywhere for the means and knowledge. When one begins to discipline his habit patterns, he finds himself inadequate and searches for guides. As water finds its own level, similar meets similar, and when he is prepared, the aspirant meets the great ones who have been treading the path of discipline and light.

It is a false notion that one has to renounce the world to practice this science. Of course one has to learn to organize oneself—but not necessarily to renounce. A day comes when an aspirant realizes that renunciation and selfless service are actually one and the same. Then he knows that living in the world and remaining unaffected, or leaving the world and becoming a renunciate, both have one and the same aim— and there is not much difference between the two.

Most of the people in the world are not aware of their capacity and ability, and have hardly any self-confidence that they can ever attain the purpose of life. But those who have acquired self-determination start practicing systematically. How to begin the practice? First, the environment should be made conducive. Then you should regulate your dietary habits and appetites. As diet seems to play an important role in life, so also do other appetites, such as sleep, sex, and self-preservation. Yoga science says, "Neither he who does not sleep nor he who sleeps too much; neither he who works too much nor he who does not work—none of these can be adepts at yoga."

The physical body needs attention so that it remains a healthy instrument for carrying out the research efficiently. Awareness of diet and exercise should become a part of one's life. In the course of study one finds that it is not only food that sustains life on this planet, but that *prana*, the vital force that we inhale, is more important than the prana from the food we eat. Of course we receive prana through food, but the quantity and quality of that prana which we receive from food alone is not enough to help the human being to live and grow. The air we breathe becomes a means of supplying the vital force, and that is how we live. It is true that breath is life.

The ancient yogis discovered various subtle breathing exercises and understood the body/breath/mind relationship in a profound and comprehensive way. The exercises explained in this book are based on the scriptures and the teachings of those great ones whom I visited in my childhood and youth. I have no reason to doubt the authenticity of these exercises, but let me frankly say that I have met many practitioners, but only a few adepts. For the convenience of advanced seekers and aspirants I have given a few exercises which are not difficult to practice, but again, I don't find that modern students have the patience, self-confidence, and self-discipline to continue the practice.

In every human heart and mind there is a constant battle between knowing the truth and enjoying the world. Many aspirants would like to practice, but only a few begin the journey, and among those few, only a fortunate few continue on. Rarely, a very fortunate few attain the goal. It is useless to brood on who is enlightened and who is not: "One who claims to be enlightened is surely not, and one who practices and follows the path may be enlightened." No one knows. It is better to practice oneself and tread the path of light.

The aspirant becomes aware that the physical body is an essential tool, but not the whole of his being, and that the breath is the life force. When he learns this, he tries to coordinate them and to understand their relationship to the thinking and feeling principles of the human mind and heart. Our search is from the gross body to the subtler realms of our being. Our thinking seldom remains under our control. A vast literature is available on the mind and its functioning, on feelings and emotions—but practical exercises for gaining control over the mind and the emotions are seldom available. This book is not an analysis of the mind, the thinking process, or the emotions. It provides specific practices for maintaining a healthy body, serene breath, and a tranquil mind, which help one to attain the goal of life. Students who are already practicing desire deeper experiences on the path. With that view in mind, this book comes into existence.

I warn all the students, readers, and aspirants not to practice any exercise explained in this book without a competent teacher. This book is written for advanced students only.

During my wanderings in India and my travels in Japan and eastern Europe I came across many astrologers, meditators, and clairvoyants. I have no reason to condemn their professional abilities, but it is true that none of them knew the science of *svarodaya*, without which one cannot have a systematic approach or access to intuitive knowledge. I have not met any astrologer who could accurately predict another's future, or even his own. Without the knowledge of svarodaya, no one could convince me about the predictive part of astrology. I have met only three people who could accurately say things about the future, for they knew the way of transcending the limiting conditions of the mind: time, space, and causation. The way of svarodaya is a systematized and organized method of gaining intuitive knowledge. I don't claim that intuitive knowledge cannot be received in other ways, but I am fully convinced that svarodaya is one method through which one can have access to the infinite library of intuition.

This book is a small part of a bulky manuscript which was written when I lived with my gurudeva in the Himalayas. For many years this manuscript remained unpublished, but my close associates and students constantly urged me to publish this book. There are five chapters in this book, which I am sure will be useful for advanced students. These chapters include information on diet and practical exercises on breath, pranayama, meditation, svarodaya, and kundalini.

I have not gone into the details of the philosophical aspects of this science, but have focused on explaining the exercises mentioned in the scriptures. I have personally examined many of the practices explained in this book. A few I have not been able to, because of the time factor—I had to leave for Japan and the Western world. But as far as I am concerned I have no doubt about the authenticity and efficacy of all these practices.

I always aspired to do extensive research on these exercises. We have set up a laboratory for examining certain breathing exercises, but so far nothing has come into my vision regarding ways to examine *dhyana* (meditation) and kundalini practices. I have not been able to accomplish my prime purpose for coming to the West because there is no laboratory with equipment sophisticated enough to help me scientifically examine and verify meditation and kundalini exercises.

I have been facing a serious difficulty: either I meet material scientists, or I meet religionists and philosophers—but I don't meet aspirants who are prepared to evaluate and verify the effects of these practices. I hope that one day this science will be popular and available for the true seekers in modern society.

The majority of people view yoga only as a system of physical culture. Very few understand that yoga science is complete in itself, and deals systematically with body, breath, mind, and spirit. When one understands that a human being is not only a physical being but a breathing being and a thinking being too, then his research does not limit itself to the body and breath only. For him, gaining control over the mind and its modifications, and the feelings and emotions, becomes more important than practicing a few postures or breathing exercises. Meditation and contemplation alone can help the aspirant in understanding, controlling, and directing the mind.

Breath and mind are close associates, which constantly influence and affect each other. Practicing pranayama helps the aspirant to control the mind, and practicing meditation helps one to fathom the deeper dimensions of life. The meditation exercises explained in this book are the exercises of concentration, and if pursued faithfully and regularly, lead one to deeper meditative states. Meditation is a conscious way of controlling the outgoing tendency of the mind, making it one-pointed and inward, and attaining perfect silence. When the mind is trained to be calm and quiet, then the aspirant attains *samadhi*, the deepest state of meditation.

When the aspirant learns to practice a meditative posture regularly and punctually, he finds certain obstacles in calming the mind. This can be because of the environment in which he lives, his food habits, unsteady posture, irregular breathing, or the unruliness of his mind. When he gains mastery of the meditative posture, making it steady, and then learns to practice pranayama, the mind still remains a barrier for him. It should be understood that *sushumna* application is the only methodical way of preventing the dissipation of the mind. When sushumna is applied, the mind finds delight in the practice of meditation. Dhyana becomes easy and spontaneous. I have described here a few methods of changing the flow of the breath and applying sushumna.

By practicing meditation the aspirant acquires the ability to pursue the awakening of kundalini. Without awakening kundalini, the individual remains primitive, unaware of the goal of life. There are many practices mentioned in the scriptures; a competent teacher imparts the knowledge of awakening this dormant force. The aspirant leads this force to the *sahasrara chakra* and accomplishes the goal of life. For the awakening of kundalini one should have the knowledge of the chakras in all their profundity. A brief description of the chakras is given in this book.

I hope that this book will inspire advanced aspirants so that they continue their practice.

chapter one

PREPARATION FOR ADVANCED PRACTICES IN PRANAYAMA

The techniques of *pranayama* are unique and can be of great benefit to the aspirants treading the path of light. These methods are highly effective and their efficacy may be fully appreciated by only the advanced students. Most often beginners focus their attention either on the yoga postures or the meditative techniques, without understanding the importance of the pranayama exercises, which affect the whole being. When one has been doing the more basic breathing exercises for some time, then he realizes that the breathing exercises are as important as the exercises of concentration or meditation. At this point the aspirant may then begin to seriously and faithfully practice pranayama and study this system.

To understand the purpose and goals of practicing pranayama it is useful to begin by looking at the meaning of the word itself. *Prana* means "breath" and *yama* means "pause." Pranayama is the means of properly regulating the otherwise irregular and hurried respiratory process without using excessive force or restraint. Pranayama regulates the three processes of exhalation *(rechaka)*, suspension *(kumbhaka)*, and inhalation *(puraka)*, and establishes control over prana, the vital force of the body. A unit of pranayama consists of inhaling to one's capacity, suspending the breath for as long as possible, and then exhaling until the lungs are empty.

Pranayama is one of the most important practices of yoga science. One of the aims of pranayama is to allow the aspirant to gain control over the nervous system. The gradual control of the nervous system then enables one to control the mind and prana, the vital energy. Pranayama is also a process intended to help one remain unaffected by disturbing thoughts and to keep the body and mind well conditioned and in perfect health.

There are many practices for the well-being of the physical body, but few individuals understand the practices that influence and transform the inner and more subtle functions of the body. The purposes of pranayama are to balance the vital principles, to bring the mind under volitional control, and to direct the vital force through certain channels in the body. These practices help reveal a subtle aspect of life and nature that can be experienced in no other way.

In *mantra yoga, laya yoga,* and *raja yoga,* the practice of pranayama is only ancillary and not of central importance; the breath is often left to find its own balance. However, in *hatha yoga* the regulation of the breath is the chief means used to achieve the goal shared by all branches of yoga.

The student who wants to practice breathing exercises must be practical in establishing a foundation and must train the body to cooperate. He must examine how he lives, the kind of food he eats, the air he breathes, his mental attitude, and how these interact. The aspirant who seeks to advance in pranayama should strive for balance.

CREATING THE PROPER ENVIRONMENT

A sincere aspirant needs solitude. The first essential in the practice of both pranayama and meditation is a quiet place where one can be by oneself. The most desirable retreat is a small, uncluttered chamber or room with fresh air, free from external disturbances. It does not matter whether this is a quiet room in one's home, a retreat in the woods, or a cubicle in a monastery, so long as it provides peace and quiet. The room should be airy and neither too cold nor too hot.

Good-quality air is essential for yoga practices, especially intensive pranayama. Cleansing and purifying the system are important aspects of the breathing practices. If the air is polluted this is not possible—in fact the ill effects of contaminated air can be compounded through increased respiration. In addition to the absence of pollution, two other properties of the air are important: its temperature and humidity. Humid air can create lethargy and indifference. Overly warm air is debilitating, while air that is too cold produces disruptive disturbances in pranic flow.

In ancient times aspirants had a small cave with a pool of water nearby. The cave was about six feet square and had a low narrow passage for an entrance. By using a cave for their practices, aspirants eliminated distracting surface conditions and noises; quietness prevailed. If, however, one is accustomed to a restless, noisy life, he may initially experience such a retreat as dull and boring, and may soon give up his practices. Therefore one should begin moderately to eliminate distractions without abruptly changing his life. He should select the most advantageous site and resolve to practice diligently.

In addition to the physical environment there is also an interpersonal environment to be reckoned with. To progress in one's practices it is preferable to live a quiet life rather than indulging in excessive companionship with the petty and worldly-minded. While ultimately the aspirant will be able to be refractory to the distractions created by the social and emotional demands of those around him, they may initially prove to be disabling. This does not necessarily mean one must separate himself from all human contact in order to practice advanced yoga.

It does mean he must carefully watch his use of energy within relationships so that he does not drain himself and thus sabotage his own efforts. One should not mix excessively with others, for such contact leads to attraction and repulsion, promotes jealousy, and arouses various sorts of unsettling emotions that will follow him to his retreat and disturb his mind. However, the company of those who are sincere and devoted to their own practice of yoga not only can prevent such negative effects, but can actually be supportive and helpful.

Association with sincere teachers and students has always been regarded as a useful adjunct to yoga practice. Either this may be found in a community of seekers, or a husband and wife may work together to create a home environment that provides such support. In order to strengthen self-discipline, one should associate with wise people in whom discipline is firmly rooted. Studying and reflecting on insightful and inspiring teachings is also helpful.

It is preferable to practice in a place free from external distractions. The aspirant is then able to search for true happiness within. One should practice according to his capacity and not try to go beyond that. In the beginning one should examine his capacity carefully and hold to a conservative limit at each practice until it becomes comparatively easy, and then he may increase the amount of practice step by step.

One should not be absorbed in thoughts of external objects, but should remain free from all of the anxieties of the world. Hallucinations, superstitions, and negative thinking should also be avoided. Control of mind, action, and speech should be practiced. Enlightening thoughts should be encouraged. One should not allow his mind to be dissipated in idle conversation and thinking. Excessive talking wastes prana and depletes one's energy. One's actions should be exact and purposeful. Let the aspirant conquer sorrow, grief, pain, and disappointment through contemplation. He will then have increased energy with which to work toward his goal.

An important aim of yoga is to accumulate and conserve every ounce of vitality possible. Until one's vital energy reaches a certain level, he will not progress to the stage of yoga that brings the greatest rewards. If the aspirant is married, the relationship can be helpful to his practice if the partners share common goals and understand and support each other. A relationship without understanding will hinder spiritual growth.

Sexual energy can distract the aspirant if it is not handled carefully. Too much sexual involvement can lead one to a slothful way of life. For the married couple, abandoning sex totally can lead to repression and suppression, which are equally harmful. The aspirant should not allow himself to be distracted so that he forgets the goal and purpose of his spiritual practices. Renunciates vigorously practice a method that is called "upward traveling" *(urdhva retas)*. In ancient times devoted students were given such practices. This practice includes *siddhasana, maha mudra, kapalabhati,* and a method of concentration that enables the student to direct his energy toward his spiritual goal, avoiding sexual indulgence. This practice is done in an austere atmosphere, with the guidance of an accomplished yogi. Only committed renunciates make efforts to practice upward traveling. Many of them fail. Only the rare, fortunate ones succeed.

Whether they are renunciates or lead a normal house-holder's life, all students should remember that food, sex, sleep, and self-preservation are the main primitive foun-tains that need to be understood and regulated so that they do not deviate from their path. Each of these urges has an equally powerful impact on the human body and mind. There should be a balance in regulating these urges. Students need to give equal attention to the regulation of each of these urges rather than to give excessive attention to any one of these drives.

The body is continually undergoing changes caused by one's own habits and actions, climate, environment, food, heat, cold, moisture, and other influences beyond the realm of human control. These continually changing phys-ical circumstances affect one's mental state. At times the mind becomes restless and it cannot be made quiet and at-tentive. The mind may also give rise to chains of thought that are totally foreign to the natural temperament of the individual and make him question his sanity.

If negative thoughts enter the mind, one should not use willpower to drive them away. Doing so only dissipates one's energy and defeats his purpose. The greater the effort one makes to drive negative thoughts away, the more they return with redoubled force. Be indifferent and quiet, and the disturbing thoughts will soon pass away. One should not be anxious about such negative thought patterns. They are natural to everyone because of the life one lives and the ex-ternal influences that affect us. The negative mental condi-tion will pass away by itself if no special attention is given to it, and soon the mind will again return to normal function-ing. Then yoga may be taken up and practiced as strenu-ously as possible within one's individual capacity.

One should practice according to his own capacity and not try to go beyond it. In the beginning one should examine his capacity carefully and hold to a conservative limit at each practice, until it becomes comparatively easy, and then the amount of practice can gradually be increased. Yoga should not be practiced to a point of tiredness or weariness. Always seek to develop and maintain a state of freshness in the body and mind during yogic practices.

Yoga practices for the body may begin at any time of the year, but the practice of pranayama should begin either in the fall months (September, October, or November) or during the spring months (February, March, or April), when the climate is moderate. One should never begin the practice of pranayama in the extreme hot, cold, or rainy seasons. Certain diseases are prone to arise in the body if one begins in the winter or in the extremes of heat or cold. In very warm weather the night hours can be used for practicing pranayama.

In the spring and autumn the air is pure. Changes in the air greatly affect the motion and functions of the human body, and thus the vigor and clarity of the mind are also affected. When the sky is serene and clear and the weather is temperate, then the body is vigorous, active, and strong, and one tends to be enthusiastic and lively.

When the weather is cloudy, foggy, and rainy, the body is languid and heavy, and one tends to be lethargic. When the temperature is rising and the air is cool and serene, the body is more robust and the appetite is stronger. Dry, pure, cool weather renders the body more active and sprightly because it strengthens the fibers and leads to better motion of the body fluids. A moist, cold air is more detrimental to health than dry air, for it makes the motion of these fluids slow and heavy; it closes the pores, relaxes the tone of the body fibers, and slows the blood. Intense cold stagnates and obstructs the fine vessels of the head, lungs, and joints. A moist, foggy atmosphere that lasts for a lengthy period, like that around lakes or marshes, creates morbidity.

In autumn's thick, cloudy, rainy weather, when there is a southerly wind and life is sedentary, with long hours of sleep, one's excretions, especially perspiration, are impeded and the pulse becomes slow, soft, and weak. During the winter the pulse is hard and strong. In May it becomes strong and forceful, and in midsummer the pulse becomes quicker but not so strong. Thus one will find that a healthy environment and the proper climate make the practice of pranayama more effective.

DIETARY CONSIDERATIONS

Though advanced yoga practices focus on internal research, in order for this work to be successful it is important that externals, such as the condition of the environment and the physical body, be set in order. Disturbing influences in the physical environment, whether they are within the body or in the world around oneself, can disrupt attempts to make progress with inner work. Disturbances in the environment or discomforts in the body draw one's consciousness to the gross physical level, and undermine his attempts to involve himself in the advanced practices of yoga.

Diet is a particularly common stumbling block for those who are attempting to tread the path of yoga, especially in the advanced stage. In order for the physical body and the nervous system to be well-tuned instruments in the pursuit of higher consciousness, food intake must be carefully and skillfully regulated. Carelessly taking too much, too little, or the wrong kind of food can disrupt both physiological and psychological functioning. Especially in the earlier steps along the path of yoga, the quality of one's consciousness is severely limited by the condition of the nervous system. The clarity and efficiency of the nervous system is constantly being affected by the way one eats.

Foods that may be quite adequate or even optimal for normal functioning in the outside world may not be conducive to creating the internal conditions that must prevail for the practice of advanced yoga techniques. A diet that is ideal for good health and psychological well-being in someone who is actively engaged in a conventional life of work and relationships may not be suitable for certain intensive practices. For this reason it must be remembered that dietary suggestions mentioned in yoga texts often apply only to specific practices and are not to be confused with general dietary recommendations that are made for the average person functioning in the busy world of everyday life.

The same principles apply to the quantity of food taken. Eating in proper measure is extremely important. This does not mean, however, that one routinely decreases the intake of food as much as possible. In fact, a diminished intake can often be counterproductive. Too little nourishment can weaken the system and undermine the capacity for carrying out the demanding and sometimes rigorous exercises involved in advanced yoga. On the other hand, too much food can be equally problematic. The heaviness and lethargy that follow even the slightest overeating will totally eliminate the possibility of performing many of the practices that are recommended in this book. The intake of food should be carefully gauged to correspond to a number of variables.

The first of these is the time of day. Ideally the major food intake should occur near the middle of the day, when the body is geared to maximal digestion. During the afternoon the movement of prana is such that alertness is decreased anyhow, and this is an appropriate time to devote to processing and assimilating nourishment. The next important factor that affects the timing of food intake is the nasal cycle. Generally, solid foods should be taken when the right nostril is flowing, while liquids are best handled when the breath is flowing in the left.

Another critical factor which affects the timing of meals, as well as the quantity of food taken, is the stage in which one finds himself with a given practice. What may be an appropriate amount of food or an appropriate time for meals during the early stages of a certain practice may no longer be appropriate as one advances. The total amount of food may be gradually decreased, and certain liquids may be substituted for some of the meals. Doing this prematurely can weaken one and undermine progress rather than facilitate it.

It is because of such misuse that the process of fasting is often damaging and ill advised. For those who are unprepared, fasting can be debilitating and a mere exercise in egoism. On the other hand, fasting is necessary at the appropriate stage of certain practices to allow the desired effects to take place.

As a general principle, allowing sufficient time between meals (when nothing is taken except perhaps liquids that are quickly assimilated) creates a number of "mini-fasts," or times when the body is not preoccupied with digestion and assimilation. It is at such times that consciousness is most unencumbered and most free to focus on breathing or to soar to those heights for which the practitioner aspires. With this in mind, it is obvious that the practice of eating between meals must be strictly eliminated in order to involve oneself in the effective practice of advanced yoga.

The system of ayurveda analyzes three vital principles, or *doshas*, that influence the body. These are *vata* (or the air-like principle), *pitta* (the fire-like principle), and *kapha* (the heavy, substantial principle). One must maintain an equilibrium among these energies. If one of the vital principles or doshas (vata, pitta, or kapha) becomes distorted, then, according to its quality, it will create some kind of problem or imbalance in the body. The effects of specific foods at various levels of practice are considered below.

Ghee

The use of *ghee*, or clarified butter, plays an important role in the diets prescribed for a number of the more rigorous yoga practices. From the perspective of ayurvedic medicine, ghee is unique: it is said to cure vatic disturbances, to diminish pitta, and to supply and replenish kapha. It also has a cooling effect. Because of this unique combination of characteristics it is particularly well suited to the conditions that prevail during rigorous pranayama. The often drastic shifts in breath and pranic flow must be prevented from creating disruptive and distracting disturbances in *vayu*, the air element. Because of its ability to "cure vata," ghee has a soothing effect that facilitates the smooth regulation of pranic flow.

The heat that is generated during the practice of pranayama can sometimes be extreme. This presents the risk of vitiating (increasing in an undesirable fashion) pitta, the fire-like principle in the body. Pitta, which corresponds closely to the *tejas tattva*, the fire element, can easily become destructive when exaggerated and uncontrolled. Among all the foodstuffs, ghee is renowned for its ability to subdue and control pitta, and for this reason it becomes extremely important in the practice of intensive pranayama, where the production of fire within is a necessary and desirable part of the basic process.

The destructive effects of excessive heat and the exaggeration of the fire-like principle in the body can actually burn away body substance and create a wasting effect if not properly regulated and controlled. The strengthening and replenishing properties of ghee, which are reflected in its capacity to increase kapha, become extremely important in preventing this burning away or wasting effect that can result from rigorous pranayama.

Milk

Of course milk has many of the same properties as ghee, since it also contains butterfat. In fact, many dietary prescriptions for advanced practices specify "rich milk," emphasizing the importance of the presence of butterfat. While many fats and oils are available and are possibilities for the diet, butterfat is unique in that it is provided by nature as the optimal fat for building and sustaining the body. Many of the same principles that hold for the use of ghee also apply to milk, though it provides, in addition to the butterfat, a well-balanced source of protein, vitamins, and minerals. One might say that milk is designed by nature to provide the most nutrition with the least expenditure of energy in digestion and assimilation. In this way nature facilitates the growth of the infant, so as to ensure the continuity of the species. The yogi capitalizes on these principles by using milk as a form of nourishment that will provide the least diversion of the body's energy or distraction of his consciousness while he pursues his advanced practices.

The most common complaint about milk as a food is its tendency to produce mucus. This effect is due to the fact that milk is primarily a body-building food—appropriately so, since it is designed for the use of infants. When taken by adults who are not building bodies, of course, but merely sustaining them, its constructive matter is not used. This accumulates and is often discharged as mucus. But during the intensive practice of pranayama this is unlikely to be a problem, because the amount of nourishment that is taken is minimal and because there is a tendency for the fire created by the practice to "burn away" matter. In such a situation the properties of milk become an asset rather than a liability.

Wheat

Grains often comprise the bulk of a person's diet. This is appropriate, since they are probably the most ideal source of carbohydrate. Their combination of certain types of fiber, vitamins, minerals, and protein, with generous proportions of carbohydrate and little fat, is well handled by the body. Carbohydrate is the most ideal fuel for the body since it burns with no residue. Of all the grains known to mankind there are two which are predominantly favored: rice and wheat.

When a choice is available, wheat is often favored. Wheat has some unique properties. It is a stimulant and therefore also potentially an irritant. It is common among yogis, who are sensitive to the effects of foods, to abstain periodically from wheat (one year in seven, for example). Some of the disadvantages of wheat can be reduced by exposing it to extreme heat. Traditionally in the East this is done by grinding it and making it into flat bread *(chapatis);* the thin layers of wheat flour are thoroughly exposed to a hot cooking surface. Wheat prepared in this way seems better tolerated than that taken as loaf breads. During intensive pranayama the heat generated within the body serves to neutralize the negative effects of the wheat, so one can benefit from its positive attributes.

Sugar

An even more concentrated form of carbohydrate is sugar. Pure cane sugar is considered an ideal food during certain advanced yoga practices. Yet sugar is often considered to be one of the major problems in an average person's diet, and beginning yoga students are cautioned against its use. Though at first blush this might seem to be a contradiction, it is not. There is, again, a marked difference between what is appropriate at one stage and at another, later, stage of practice. Sugar is almost pure carbohydrate. Carbohydrate is simply trapped energy. It is formed when a reaction involving carbon dioxide and water creates a sort of hydrated carbon and releases oxygen. The reaction is endo-energetic: that is, it takes up energy, in this case, energy from the sun. The metabolism of this carbohydrate (breaking it back down into carbon dioxide and water by recombining it with oxygen) releases the sun's energy inside the body.

In the case of starch, the carbohydrate is composed of chains of sugar molecules which break off successively, releasing a steady output of energy. With sugar, or simple carbohydrate, there is a massive availability of energy at once. Just as the unprepared student is incapable of constructively handling the overwhelming surges of energy produced when he prematurely performs certain pranayama exercises, so also is he unable to deal with the surges of energy from metabolized sugar until he reaches certain levels of accomplishment. Thus a moderate intake of sugar is recommended during the practice of advanced techniques, while it is recommended that it be much more limited in the average diet. Sugar intake in those who are not engaged in intensive practices can produce drastic irregularities in energy flow (hypoglycemic and hyperglycemic episodes) with consequent mental and emotional upheavals.

Fruit

Fruits are high-sugar foods and many of the considerations that apply to sugar apply to them, too. They are also rich sources of vitamins and minerals, and as such offer not only fuel but a generous supply of the nutrients that are needed to burn that fuel well. The yogi utilizes nutrients to their utmost, since his metabolism is functioning at a peak of efficiency during his practices. Still, at least until the most advanced stages, the yogi needs certain nutrients in his food. Even in reasonably good-quality food these nutrients are often damaged to some extent by age, exposure to air, or deterioration due to heat. To the extent that the complex molecules of food are damaged, the food has a devitalizing, *tamasic,* effect. To the extent that the original vitality of the plant ingredients has been lost, the food also has an increased tamasic effect. Fruit is especially suited to the yogic diet since it is taken fresh and live, and yet is light and easy to digest.

Foods to Avoid

Meat and processed, packaged, and fermented foods are, of course, proscribed since they all have strongly tamasic effects. Flesh foods not only have lost their vitality through death (and often intentional aging), but they also stimulate the aggressive and instinctual energies of the lower chakras. Though certain schools of yoga have devised approaches to transmute these energies, arousing them during most practices is simply a disruption and a distraction.

While diets for yoga practices may vary, and specific prescriptions are sometimes given, in general such diets may be thought of as falling into three basic stages:

Diet During Beginning Levels of Practice. Normally this is a balanced vegetarian diet, based on grains with legumes *(dahl),* fresh-cooked green vegetables, fresh milk products, and fresh, raw fruit. Ghee is used sparingly as a cooking medium, and a variety of seasonings and spices may also be used, but harsher spices, such as chili peppers, raw onions, or garlic, are avoided.

Diet During Intermediate Levels of Practice. At this level, diet will be based on specific grains, usually wheat and barley, that are often fried in ghee with mild spices such as ginger, and which may be cooked with sugar. Legumes are used less frequently and may be restricted to fresh (not dried) beans such as chana (similar to garbanzos). Fruits and milk play an increasing role.

Diet During Advanced Intensive Practice. When advanced practices are being done, most solid foods are dropped, though fresh fruits may still be taken in moderation. Milk, especially that rich in butterfat, becomes the focal point of the diet, and is taken, as always, after boiling. It may be combined with water, spices, or sugar. Specific dietary recommendations made later in this book should be considered as being specific to those individuals who are doing advanced pranayama under the guidance of a teacher, and are not intended for general use.

REGULATION OF THE BREATH

With the regulation of the breath, karma acquired both in this life and in the past may be burnt up. Just as a fire consumes a heap of timber, it is said that pranayama makes the mind free from all illusion. As fire, which is a latent potential of wood, does not become potent except by friction, so also wisdom, which is already latent within each person, reveals itself through pranayama practice. It is said in the texts that through pranayama the power of levitation is acquired, diseases are cured, spiritual energy is awakened, calmness and mental powers are obtained, and the practitioner is filled with bliss. When one develops control over the sympathetic system through the practice of pranayama, he becomes the master of his body; he can cast off his body at will. If one practices pranayama continuously for a year, he is sure to attain wisdom. Pranayama is a basic step on the path of enlightenment.

The first goal of these breathing exercises is to control the *prana vayu*, so that the disturbing forces arising from within are eliminated and the mind becomes focused and one-pointed. Later the entire involuntary system is made voluntary. Voluntary control leads the aspirant to a state of samadhi.

One must understand what is meant by vayu—its qualities and attributes. The word *vayu* has no exact equivalent in the English language, so it must be defined at some length. It literally means "that which flows." It is the agent for all motion. Without this medium, no motion can be manifested and one cannot express anything. In breathing exercises, it is vayu that one seeks to control.

An analogy may make this a little clearer. All phenomena are said to be motion or vibration. This implies something to vibrate—a medium or a vehicle. Motion has as its constituent parts motion and pause, for where one finds motion, one always finds a pause or cessation. These concepts are expressed in Sanskrit by the terms *shakti, vayu,* and *karma.* Unless these three things are combined, there is no vibration. There must be an impulse (shakti, or energy) that produces motion, a medium of action (vayu), and a force of resistance that restrains motion (karma). The power or impulse behind vayu is shakti, energy; the obstruction in the path of shakti is karma. Karma produces the pause of vayu. Animation or vibration is affected according to the strength of these factors. If karma is greater, then the pause will be greater, and the motion will be less. If one sets his mind to a task but the circumstances prevent it, then karma is stronger than shakti or vayu.

Another analogy is used in the tantric exposition. Consider the human being as a water system in which our shakti, our inclination toward self-realization, is the pressure on the system; vayu, the medium, is water; and karma, our limiting quality, is the pipe. If our inclination or the pressure (shakti) is greater than our environmental resistance (or the pipe's size), a greater volume of vayu can move through the pipe. If the pressure (shakti) is great enough and the pipe is weak enough, the volume of vayu will burst the pipe: if one's shakti is strong enough, the bondage and limitations of his karma can be overcome. It can be seen, therefore, that the conditions determining vibrations are various. When the motion is greater and the resistance weaker, shakti is the ruling unit. When there is greater intensity of flow, vayu is stronger.

From the ayurvedic perspective, shakti is considered to be the potentiality of all energy, and vayu to be kinetic energy. As pointed out in the discussion of diet, vayu or vata is considered to be one of the three doshas, or vital principles, the others being pitta (the principle of heat) and kapha (the principle of heaviness and substance). Vayu is that which contracts, expands, provides pressure, and moves, connecting all the other forces and making it possible for them to work. Excessive, intense, or extended action of vayu generates disease, and the weakening of vayu is the cause of certain kinds of fever. We understand the character of vayu by observing sounds, the blood flow, symptoms such as the hair standing on end, throbbing of the temples, gooseflesh, twitching, flashes of light, noises in the stomach and bowels, the cracking of the joints, sneezing, hiccoughing, the quality of cutting or shooting pains, and other signs. If the body shakes or trembles while one is practicing hatha yoga, it indicates that vayu is strong and the process must be slowed down. Due to vayu, a human being wanders in the cycle of births and deaths, but the yogi seeks to be free from this cycle and therefore perseveres in his practices.

Vayu is the medium through which any desire, inclination, or motion works, and has forty-nine varieties. The vehicle of these forty-nine varieties of vayu is air. Vayu is like a rider, whereas air is like the horse. We know the quality of air by its effects, and our various senses reveal its existence to us. In the same manner we detect and know vayu inside the body. Vayu gives us the sense of feeling, for without vayu our tactile sense is inactive: the lack of sensation in a paralyzed part of the body is evidence of the absence of vayu.

The action of vayu eliminates or throws off waste material from the body. Vayu is also the power of digestion and is the basis of the reduction of food into energy by the different parts of the digestive system. The glands have vayu in them, and it is through vayu that they ingest the essence of food. The vayu in the body corresponds to both the cerebrospinal and sympathetic nervous systems. Control over vayu means the practical control of the cerebrospinal system over the sympathetic system. It is the purpose of pranayama to bring these vayus under control. Thus the main vayus will be explained in greater detail in chapter three.

Through modern chemistry we know about the physical composition of air (oxygen, hydrogen, nitrogen, and carbon dioxide), but in the science of pranayama we study other factors, such as the resistance, functions, and energies of air.

ASPECTS OF THE BREATH

As noted earlier, exhalation is called rechaka in Sanskrit; inhalation is known as puraka; and suspension of the breath is kumbhaka. Pranayama signifies the control of these operations. When one can suspend his respiratory movements for five minutes and twenty-four seconds, he is considered to be an adept at pranayama. Then he can perceive the existence of the universal life force within. It is claimed in the texts that after five minutes of suspension, the brain requires six hours to return to its former state.

The physical aspect of pranayama is divided into two stages. In the first, the suspension of breath (kumbhaka) is associated with inspiration and expiration. That is, kumbhaka is timed with rechaka and puraka. In the second case, suspension is done alone without inspiration or expiration, and kumbhaka is sustained for as long as the aspirant wishes. This, of course, is done only when one has become an expert in the first stage.

The physical effects of suspension are exercised nerves, the equalization of inhalation and exhalation, the reduction of the weight of the body, and a decrease in the speed of thoughts. Since the period of each thought is lengthened, there is time to fully comprehend and analyze it. A thought can be made to remain before the mind for seconds, whereas its normal speed is two twenty-fifths of a second.

Ida and *pingala*, situated on each side of the spinal column, are joined at a point deep behind the forehead, at the *ajna chakra* (eyebrow center), where one finds a small but significant ganglion called the ganglion of Ribes. Ida goes around this ganglion to the right and terminates in the left nostril; pingala goes around it on the left and ends in the right nostril. In passing along the posterior side of the spinal cord, those two channels change their positions several times, alternating left and right, and meet again below at the ganglion impar, located in front of the coccyx, which corresponds to the *muladhara chakra*. These channels communicate repeatedly with *sushumna* throughout its course. For example, one such meeting place corresponds to the superior hypogastric plexus.

Through the practice of kumbhaka the fibers of the vagus nerve are stimulated, and there is stimulation of the vagal center in the medulla oblongata, with a slowing of the heart's action to the point of total cessation. The vagus nerve has a more extensive distribution than any other cranial nerve. It contains both sensory and motor fibers, and it supplies both the motor and sensory nerves to the organs of speech and respiration: the pharynx, esophagus, heart, and the stomach motor fibers. Stimulation of this nerve at its center in the medulla oblongata causes the inhibition of such organs as the heart, lungs, and larynx, and the acceleration of the movement of the stomach. This vagal center is also excited by the stimulation of its fibers that end in the nasal mucous membranes, the larynx, and the lungs. *Kundalini shakti* may be excited when the vagus nerve is violently vibrated by pranayama, so that the actions of the heart and lungs are reduced to a minimum.

When one inhales he is taking in *prana,* and when he exhales he is throwing out *apana.* The more prana one takes in, the more vitality he possesses. Ordinarily our breathing habits are irregular and erratic. Thus the motion of the lungs is irregular, which affects the heart, the pumping station to the brain, and the entire metabolism is disturbed. The yogi who is capable of regulating the length of the exhalation and inhalation enjoys perfect health and acquires spiritual power. The advanced practitioner of pranayama learns to reap the same benefits by balancing and extending both exhalation and inhalation.

When practicing pranayama it is important to consciously observe the phenomena that take place when we breathe. It is necessary for one to create a certain amount of pranic pressure in the system. This pressure should be a little greater than in the normal process of respiration. This is done by inhaling a greater amount of air than normal for a certain period of time, creating an effect that will last for a longer period. The ratio between the period of inhalation and the more lasting effect of the pressure this generates is 1:60. Therefore a person who does long, deep, heavy breathing for one minute creates pressure that has an effect for one hour; that is, the value of such exercise will not be exhausted for approximately an hour. For the welfare of the individual the general rule is a practice period of 24 minutes every 24 hours, which would produce the necessary pressure. Some individuals, rather than practicing for 24 minutes at one sitting, practice for 15 minutes twice daily, morning and evening.

The mind undergoes various changes in the waking and sleeping states. At the approach of darkness, one's physical condition is naturally altered by the gathering up of the positive forces in nature. As a result, the senses sleep and receive no impressions from without. The average amount of absolute rest during a night's sleep is 11½ minutes. The remainder of the time is subject to muscular or mental action. Sleep, as a rule, has an overpowering influence on the mind due to its quality of inertia.

In yoga, the three manifestations of wakefulness, dreaming, and dreamless sleep are the results of certain temperatures at which sensory organs ordinarily work, all being under the influence of the cardiac temperature. In Sanskrit, the control of this phenomenon is called *sadhanatita*. When the negative ida current, the cold current, reaches its limit and has become predominant over the positive current, consciousness sleeps in the heart. When the positive current, pingala, reaches its daily extreme, the actions of the sensory organs are no longer synchronous with the internal modifications of the *tattvas,* and wakefulness exists in all its activity. Nature always seeks to maintain a balance in these two elements, heat and cold. When the yogi, using the power of prana or mantra, activates this cardiac temperature, he is able to bring about the results that his level of competency permits.

The Buddhists say too much sleep destroys all spiritual enthusiasm. By not yielding to the influence of sleep for a night or two, one gains strength. An occasional vigil is truly helpful. One should eliminate, step by step, the qualities of sloth, sleep, confusion, temptation, infatuation, and the sense of blankness.

The perfection of pranayama leads to a decrease in sleep and in the waste products of the body. As the dreaming person feels the lightness of his body in his dream rambles, so the aspirant finds his solid body to be as light as air. He never perspires, his semen dries up, and the seminal force ascends to come back as nectar (the *amrita* of shiva/shakti). He becomes free from disease and sorrow, and there is neither an increase nor a decrease of the vital principles. When this last result comes, he may be irregular in his diet or other practices with impunity. He may take a very large or a very small quantity of food, or no food at all.

Through pranayama one attains the power to live without air, food, or drink, as well as the power of levitation. One's mind becomes calm and blissful. There is also an exaltation of mental powers, and spiritual energy is awakened. As the impurities in metal are burnt away by fire, so the imperfections of the senses are burnt by the control of prana. With the control of prana the bodily heat, *agni,* increases daily. With the increase of agni, food will be more easily digested. When food is properly digested, *rasa,* the metabolized food essence, is increased, and with the increase of rasa, the bodily root principles, the *dhatus,* the life essences, increase. With the increase of the dhatus, wisdom increases. Thus, the imperfections of scores of years are burnt up.

There are four kinds of respiration: windy, gasping, emotional, and pure respiration. The first three are not harmonized. The breath is known as windy when it makes noise passing in and out. The second kind of respiration is broken and irregular, as if one were gasping for air. The third is without either noise or gasping, but the breath is uneven; for example, one may inhale rather quickly and exhale slowly. The last, pure respiration, is a calm, regular process, tuned to nature, with one inhalation to four beats of the heart and one exhalation to four beats of the heart.

TYPES OF KUMBHAKA AND THEIR EFFECTS

The *Hatha Yoga Pradipika* lists eight types of suspension, or kumbhaka, which result in strengthening the action of the heart valves, bringing the air closer to the blood, aiding in the exchange of gases, and creating a beneficial pressure in any unused or inflamed portions of the lungs and air passages.

Patanjali describes four types of kumbhaka. The first is called *bahya kumbhaka,* in which the breath is suspended outside the lungs. The second is called *abhyantara,* in which suspension is done with the lungs filled. The third and fourth varieties are called *kevala kumbhaka.* In the third type, when the aspirant so wishes, the breath stops suddenly of its own accord without physical effort. In the fourth type, the pause is brought about after many inhalations and exhalations, and there is no effort made to maintain suspension, as there is with the third kumbhaka.

In the beginning, as the duration of kumbhaka increases the body will grow hot and perspire freely. This perspiration should not be wiped off but should be massaged into the body, thus adding to one's strength. Then one should take a bath. In time, this excess perspiration will cease. In the intermediate stage, as progress is made and the breath comes under control, the body will quiver and possibly move on its seat.

In the third stage, one attains steadiness after the breath is made motionless. The aspirant will then be able to do things with ease that others find impossible; he will be extraordinarily strong, and pain and grief will be unknown to him. He may experience hallucinations resulting from an excited state of the nervous system. As the nervous system becomes cleansed and in proper functioning order, these visions will pass away, and the mind will settle down to a more rational and intelligent state. Visions of the forms upon which one meditates are merely signs of perseverance, and they have no intrinsic value in themselves. All visions, imaginings, hallucinations, and the like should be shunned. The serious student is seeking intelligence and not disordered mental states or the experience of seeing absurd and senseless visions or symbols. In the higher stages of pranayama, flashes of truth will illuminate one's heart now and then.

The head sounds heard during the practice of pranayama are caused by the rushing of blood through the arteries and veins and may indicate congestion. When these conditions occur it is advisable to go slowly, to be more moderate in one's eating, and to practice more often, but not for so long a time at one sitting. These symptoms do not indicate any harm, but one should have reasonable regard for this condition. The noises will pass away as the *nadis* become purified. In later and more advanced practice, they will only be heard when certain pressure is created in those parts.

What is known as total suspension requires 13½ minutes and results in the experience of samadhi. It is said that the senses become suspended when one can perform kumbhaka for a period of 10 minutes 48 seconds. Though this may seem physiologically impossible, with gradual training the body can function with dramatically less oxygen due to a slowing down of its metabolic activity. When a yogi can suspend his breath for about 1½ hours, there is very little in this world that is not possible for him. A tranquil state of mind develops when respiration can be suspended for 21 minutes 30 seconds. This state may also be brought about by the use of mantra or by fixing the attention on the subtle sounds. Suspension of the breath for 2 hours 42 minutes leads one beyond time and space to a superconscious state.

When the aspirant, seated in *padmasana*, the lotus pose, can leave the ground and rise in the air, he has attained *vayu siddhi*, success over the pranas. This destroys the darkness of ignorance. As long as one has not gained this siddhi, he should not give up his practices, and should observe all the rules and restrictions laid down. By continued practice he will gain power over nature and the animals that dwell within the domain of nature, even over tigers and lions.

The first purpose in the art of pranayama is to oxygenate the blood and not allow the energy that results from oxygenation to be dissipated. The second purpose is to eliminate as much waste material as one can. Therefore one should inhale as much as possible and suspend the breath, so that there may be a more complete exchange of the gases. The third goal is to introduce pressure into the system, maintaining a proper balance between the outside and inside pressures. When this balance is not maintained, the nerves—and, in turn, the mind and muscles—are affected; the body trembles and the mind fails to function normally. This is analogous to a jar which, half-filled with water, makes noises when handled or carried. But when the jar is full and still, no sound is produced; when the body is full of pressure, one manifests determination, enthusiasm, and willpower. The fourth purpose of pranayama is the control of thoughts. In the final stage, the breath of life is made perfectly serene, followed by its passage through sushumna to the head, where knowledge of the universal life force is attained. This is followed by an understanding of the purpose of life.

chapter two

THE PRACTICE OF
PRANAYAMA

In this chapter, we will give an overview of advanced pranayama practices. We will start with the purification practices, *kapalabhati* and *nadi shodhanam,* and then go on to explain the importance of the three *bandhas,* or locks: *mula bandha* (the root lock), *uddiyana bandha* (the navel lock), and *jalandhara bandha* (the chin lock). We will also discuss the group of practices that include *surya bhedana, ujjayi, sitali, sitkari,* and *bhastrika.* Collectively, these practices lead to the awakening of sushumna.

KAPALABHATI

Kapalabhati is a breathing exercise but not a pranayama exercise in the strictest sense. It is a process of purifying the nerves and cleansing the body of kapha. It is one of the six processes of cleansing the nadis, and a practice of considerable spiritual value as well. There is no kumbhaka (breath retention) in this practice. The exercise consists of rechaka (exhalation) and puraka (retention) only, with rechaka being the principal part of the exercise and puraka supplementary.

The accomplished pose, *siddhasana*, is necessary for the practice of kapalabhati. The spine is made erect, and the hands are rested upon the knees. A vigorous practice of kapalabhati vibrates almost every tissue of the body. The body becomes more and more agitated as the exercise is continued with its original vigor until it becomes difficult to control one's posture. Thus the foot lock in siddhasana is necessary to maintain one's seat throughout the exercise.

In kapalabhati the abdominal muscles and diaphragm come into play. These are suddenly and vigorously contracted, giving an inward push to the abdominal viscera. As a result the diaphragm recedes into the thorax, expelling the air from the lungs. In normal respiration, inhalation is active and the process of exhalation is passive. In kapalabhati, rechaka and puraka are performed in quick succession with a sudden and vigorous in-stroke of the abdominal muscles during exhalation, followed by a relaxation of these muscles during inhalation. Rechaka will occupy about one-fourth the time of puraka. The relaxation during inhalation is a passive act, whereas the contraction during exhalation is a most active one.

No pause should be allowed between inhalation and exhalation until a round is completed. One should start with 11 expulsions. Generally three rounds are performed at each sitting, and two sittings are performed each day, morning and evening. Eleven expulsions may be added each week until 120 expulsions are done in each round. Those who feel able may double this number of expulsions in each round. The maximum should be three rounds of three minutes each at a sitting, but the system should not be strained to reach this goal. Between successive rounds, normal respiration is resumed to provide the necessary rest. This period of normal respiration may be varied according to one's need. From 30 to 60 seconds should be enough.

One should pay attention only to one's abdominal muscles. The attention should be focused on administering abdominal strokes against a center in the lower abdomen where the spiritual energy, kundalini, dwells. Eventually the nervous system becomes actively balanced, and one experiences first a throbbing and then a form of serene light glowing at this particular center.

As a result of this exercise great quantities of carbon dioxide are eliminated and similar amounts of oxygen are absorbed into the system. The blood is made richer, and all the tissues of the body are renewed. Kapalabhati has no equal as an exercise for enhancing oxygenation. It corrects ailments arising from cold and helps to arrest old age. It has beneficial effects on the nerves, as well as improving the circulation and metabolism.

In addition to purifying the nerves, kapalabhati is practiced to awaken certain nerve centers and to make the practice of pranayama more efficient by quieting the respiratory center. A few rounds of kapalabhati should be performed daily before doing the higher practices of pranayama. Five minutes of practice will be sufficient to induce a state of trance when one is adept in this practice.

The speed with which one performs kapalabhati should not be increased at the cost of thoroughness. Beginning with one expulsion a second, the practice may be increased to two a second; 120 per minute is a good rate for a normal person. The practice may be developed to the rate of 200 a minute, but to exceed this limit would render the expirations so shallow that they would lose their efficacy. The vigor of the expulsions should be maintained; speed should not be allowed to reduce the vigor of the abdominal contractions. The degree of vigor, the speed, the number of expulsions in a single round, the number of rounds in one sitting, and the total amount of exercise done in a day should be carefully and judiciously determined.

An Alternative Method

Pucker the lips and push them out a little. Then inhale slowly through the mouth and try to feel the air make contact with the back of the throat. When the inhalation is complete, "swallow" and suspend the breath with the pressure low in the abdomen. This practice cures indigestion and many bodily diseases, and contributes to longevity.

Breathing hard induces the *apas* and *prithivi tattvas*. (The tattvas are explained in chapter three.) It may be added that placing a tight band around the right arm above the elbow and around the right thigh above the knee also excites these tattvas, especially prithivi.

NADI SHODHANAM

The purification of the nadis, or nerves, is the first step in the practice of pranayama. The practice of nadi shodhanam (channel purification) may be done twice daily (morning and evening); three times a day (morning, noon, and evening); four times a day (morning, noon, evening, and midnight); or at an advanced stage, eight times a day (every three hours). At a minimum it should be practiced for a period of 48 minutes twice daily and extended to four times a day as soon as the student is capable, or as close to this schedule as circumstances permit. The cleansing of the nadis by pranayama can be accomplished in three months, or in some cases much earlier.

Pranayama should not be done at a time when one is hungry, when the stomach is loaded with food, or when one is tired. Lack of moderation in diet will cause various diseases and thus prevent success. In advanced stages one should regularly practice retaining the breath. By doing so one will develop great control over his breath and eventually become able to retain the breath for as long as he wishes. Without purified nadis one cannot become accomplished in pranayama. Therefore the first aim should be to cleanse the body completely. A sound body in good health is the foundation of a sound mind.

In yoga the development of inner strength is traditionally said to be impeded by six factors: overeating; excessive exertion; acting in ways that shock the body and dissipate one's energies, such as taking a cold bath in the morning, eating at night, or eating only fruit; the excessive company of people; irregularity or unsteadiness in one's practices; and oversleeping. The last—immoderate sleep—produces sluggishness, dulls the mind, obstructs the memory, and dissipates one's physical and spiritual strength. Sleep in the daytime increases the three doshas and should be strictly avoided.

Ideally the student should rise in the morning at dawn or at about 4 a.m. With some effort, rising early will not be difficult but will become as natural as rising late. After cleansing one's teeth and emptying the bowels and bladder, one should begin his practice with yoga postures. *Sarvangasana,* the shoulderstand, should be performed last so that jalandhara bandha, the chin lock, may be done more easily. After the postures one should practice pranayama. One should not, however, practice pranayama when feeling uneasy, depressed, or dejected. After pranayama, meditation should be practiced. For meditative practice one should sit in the same place at the same time each day. The eyes should be closed and one should not stir on his seat. The body and head should be erect.

If one wants to attain the maximum benefit, it is important to be regular in his practices. Those who practice irregularly derive little benefit. One should set an initial goal of at least three months' practice so that he can form a habit and not go back to his past grooves. Good control can be developed in three months. With zeal and tenacity one can become adept in six months.

Under the direct guidance of a teacher the student can practice for 1½ hours at both sunset and midnight. As soon as one is able he should practice channel purification four times a day, doing the practice at least eight times at a sitting, and continuing the practice for at least three months. The ideal standard of practice is four times during the day: morning (4 a.m. to 6 a.m.), noon (10 a.m. to noon), evening (4 p.m. to 6 p.m.), and night (10 p.m. to midnight), until one can do 80 rounds with retention of the breath at each practice period, making 320 rounds a day. Start at 10 rounds the first day, and increase the number of rounds by 4 a day. It will take about three months to reach the maximum.

In the beginning, 36 seconds of kumbhaka is regarded as mild, and twice this, 72, is average. The final practice is three times the first, or 108, which is considered to be intense. This practice can be injurious if it is done without a guide.

There is a specific method (known as the *vishnu mudra*) that is used for closing the nostrils when practicing nadi shodhanam. The right hand is brought up to the nose, and the index and middle fingers folded so that the right thumb can be used to close the right nostril, and the ring finger used to close the left nostril. (As an alternative, the index and middle fingers, or simply the index finger, can remain relaxed at the bridge between the eyebrows.) When both nostrils are to remain open, the hand may be rested upon the knee.

There are at least three methods of basic nadi shodhanam taught to beginners to prepare them for nadi shodhanam with kumbhaka. Under the guidance of a competent teacher, kumbhaka can be integrated into any of these basic methods. The following is a description of one of these methods.

During daylight hours nadi shodhanam is begun by closing the right nostril and exhaling completely through the left. At the end of the exhalation, immediately inhale for the same length of time as the exhalation. Then close the left nostril and repeat the same exhalation and inhalation through the right nostril. This is one round of pranayama. During the night the practice begins by exhaling through the right nostril. It is important to keep the head straight throughout the practice and to breathe as silently and as smoothly as possible.

One should determine his capacity and breathe out and in as slowly as possible, counting the length of time it takes for each exhalation and inhalation and keeping them equal. With each succeeding day's practice one can extend the length of time for each breath until he is able to exhale for 16 seconds and inhale for 16 seconds.

The aspirant can then change the ratio and exhale for twice the time of the inhalation. When the aspirant can exhale for 32 seconds and inhale for 16 seconds he is ready to introduce kumbhaka. When one practices nadi shodhanam with kumbhaka, the ratio is 4:16:8. That is, the student inhales for a count of 4, retains for a count of 16, and then exhales for 8 seconds.

As practice progresses the basic ratio remains the same (1:4:2), but the length of the count itself changes as the student's capacity expands. After one can inhale for 16, retain for 64, and then exhale for 32 seconds, the period of the retention is again doubled, so the retention continues for 128 seconds.

Nadi shodhanam should always be practiced on an empty stomach. It can be practiced regularly at least one hour before eating. When one practices with retention, he will notice warmth and sweating at the forehead. One month's practice will make the eyes clear, and they will shine brightly. This practice makes the body light and strengthens the appetite. It may produce sounds in the head; if this occurs, one should stop practicing.

BANDHAS

Like other physical exercises, simple breathing exercises such as diaphragmatic breathing can be healthy and helpful. But in order to really practice pranayama, the knowledge and application of the bandhas is important. Without the application of the bandhas, pranayama practices can be injurious to one's health. A comprehensive knowledge of both the theory and practice of the bandhas is essential.

The word *bandha* literally means "to lock; to bind; to control." Bandhas are practices for unfolding, controlling, and rechanneling the finer force that is awakened through some of the vigorous pranayama exercises done by yogis. Three bandhas are the most important: mula bandha (the root lock), uddiyana bandha (the navel lock), and jalandhara bandha (the chin lock). Other locks, such as the tongue lock and the teeth lock, are also mentioned in yoga manuals, but all have a specific purpose, and are taught by teachers familiar with their effects and application.

MULA BANDHA (THE ROOT LOCK)

This bandha is performed by contracting the anal sphincter muscle forcibly and pulling it upward. Siddhasana is the best posture for the practice of this bandha, since the heel is positioned at the perineum, fixed against the center between the anus and the sex organ. This helps to maintain the bandha without excessive effort.

As a preparation for accomplishing mula bandha, the student practices *ashvini mudra,* which is done by contracting and releasing the anal sphincter muscle. After a period of time, when the student has gained some control over the muscles, mula bandha is introduced.

Because of the pressure on the anal sphincter during mula bandha, heat is generated, which causes *apana vayu* to move upward. The usual tendency of this vayu is to move downward. However, this practice forces apana to move upward and unite with *prana vayu* at the navel center.

Ultimately in the course of its upward journey the energy aroused at the base of the spine assimilates apana (at the muladhara chakra) and prana (in the region of the navel and chest), and then reaches the forehead. There, with the help of other mudras and *maha vedha kriya,* it is forced to enter into the central channel, sushumna, leaving its normal course through ida and pingala. Eventually mula bandha becomes spontaneous and effortless, although during the initial stages of *sadhana* (practice) one has to make conscious effort to perfect this bandha.

UDDIYANA BANDHA (THE NAVEL LOCK)

This bandha is practiced so that the energy that has been aroused and that is moving upward can be brought under voluntary control at the navel center. During its initial stage this bandha is practiced in a standing pose, bending slightly forward and resting the hands on the knees. With the body in this position one exhales completely, placing the chin at the hollow of the throat. While suspending the breath he then pulls up the abdominal muscles to his fullest capacity, creating a cavity in the abdomen. The position is held as long as possible and is then released. Later, when a student advances and the abdominal muscles are under his control, this bandha can be performed in any of the meditative postures.

The abdominal lift known as *agni sara* helps attain even greater control over the abdominal muscles and the pelvic region. Agni sara creates a bridge between the practice of mula bandha and uddiyana bandha. The whole area from the base of the spine to the navel center is contracted and pulled upward. At this stage uddiyana bandha is not muscular contraction alone—rather it involves the entire energy system, which is the core theme in the practice of pranayama and the awakening of kundalini. It is with the help of this exercise that a yogi unites prana and apana and makes them move upward. At its accomplishment an aspirant can overcome physical ailments caused by derangements of prana and apana.

JALANDHARA BANDHA (THE CHIN LOCK)

The chin lock is performed by bending the head forward and placing the chin at the hollow of the throat. It helps control the energy moving upward and prevents excessive pressure in the head. Thus only the amount of vital force which can be handled is allowed to reach the head; the rest of the vital force is restrained here at the throat center.

SURYA BHEDANA KUMBHAKA (THE SECRET OF THE SUN)

There are four *bhedanas* proper: surya, ujjayi, sitali, and bhastrika. Surya bhedana increases the heat of the body.

Through the process of surya bhedana the aspirant cures diseases that result from an insufficiency of oxygen. The practice rids one of pulmonary, cardiac, and liver diseases; cleanses the frontal sinuses; destroys disorders of vayu; increases the bodily heat (pitta); awakens kundalini; slows the aging process; and prevents premature death.

This exercise is a method of breathing by inhaling through the right nostril only. Inhale to full capacity through the right nostril, swallow, suspend the breath, and then do the chin lock. Maintain kumbhaka as long as possible. Then carefully exhale through the left nostril, slowly and with unbroken, continuous force. Repeat again, inhaling through the right nostril and exhaling through the left. During suspension maintain some control and tension in the abdominal muscles. Through this practice of putting pressure on the solar plexus one's mental abilities are developed. Putting pressure on any part of the trunk regulates the breathing and evaporates kapha.

This practice may be started with 10 pranayamas a day and increased daily by 5, until 80 can be done. When fully perfected, surya bhedana may be done repeatedly and kumbhaka may be maintained for as long as excessive perspiration does not burst forth from the hair roots or the fingertips.

The *Hatha Yoga Pradipika* suggests that after one inhales he should perform jalandhara, and at the end of kumbhaka he should contract the throat and pull in the navel by doing uddiyana. Through this practice kundalini is awakened and prana is forced into the *brahma nadi* (sushumna).

One may do this practice in the *siddhasana, padmasana,* or *sukhasana* postures. After practicing surya bhedana kumbhaka one should do ujjayi, sitkari, sitali, and then finally bhastrika, all of which are discussed immediately following. Other practices may also be done.

UJJAYI

The word *ujjayi* means "to lift up." This breathing exercise may be done in any pose suitable for pranayama. Before starting this practice, the tongue and mouth must be thoroughly cleansed and *khechari mudra* (curling the tongue back and tucking it in toward the palate) must be practiced until saliva permeates the mouth. Then the practice is begun. Ujjayi is a deep-chest inhalation with a slightly closed glottis, followed by suspension; then one exhales slowly. This practice increases the heat of the body. In ujjayi the breath is drawn in through both nostrils, by partially closing the glottis and by expanding the chest, making a sound like sobbing of a low, sweet, and uniform pitch. The abdominal muscles are controlled by a very slight contraction that is maintained throughout the inhalation. The entire inhalation must be slow, smooth, and uniform, so that no friction at all takes place in the nostrils. The walls of the chest should stand firm with elevated ribs, for only then can the glottis do its work. When the inhalation is complete, one swallows the breath, followed by kumbhaka and jalandhara. A slight contraction of the upper abdomen is carefully maintained, and the real benefits of the kumbhaka lie in this contraction. Kumbhaka should not be held to a point of suffocation, nor should it prevent a smooth, proportionate exhalation.

Exhalation is done through either the left nostril or through both nostrils, with the glottis partially closed, producing a sound of low, uniform pitch. At no time should control of the breath be lost. From the beginning of rechaka the abdominal muscles should undergo a continual contraction, until the chest contracts completely, thus expelling the very last portion of air in the lungs without strain. The length of this exhalation should be about twice that of the inhalation. Seek to prolong the duration of the inhalation and exhalation during each round. Initially about four rounds a minute is an adequate effort. Never should the exhalation be prolonged to such an extent that one cannot proceed with the next round without gasping for additional breath. The mind may be focused on the breath at the glottis, where it meets with friction, and concentration should be kept there during kumbhaka, or one may picture the air passing to and from the kundalini as a thin, luminous vapor.

After the practice period is finished, if one is not excessively tired, the breath that fills the mouth should be swallowed and taken to the region of the solar plexus. There a sort of belching act is done, without opening the nostrils or mouth. Next allow the air to rise and then make it go down again. This aids in awakening all the nadis from the throat to the navel and is a practice of great help when kundalini begins to rise up.

As a preliminary step, a week or so may be devoted to uj-jayi, leaving off kumbhaka. This preparatory exercise can be practiced at any time, whether standing, walking, or sitting.

One should begin ujjayi with 7 rounds, adding 3 rounds to each sitting every week, according to one's individual capacity. The maximum number of rounds performed daily should be 320, distributed over two to four sittings, although 240 rounds are sufficient for physical health. Once this practice is perfected one is never subject to diseases originating from kapha such as indigestion, dysentery, consumption, cough, fever, enlarged spleen, or nervous disorders.

SITKARI

Sitkari keeps the body cool. It is best to do this practice at night, taking a glass of warm milk 20 to 30 minutes before beginning. Start by keeping the teeth closed and the tongue fixed so that it does not touch the palate, the bottom of the mouth, or the teeth. Firmly pressing the teeth together, draw air through the mouth, making as much noise as possible, and pull from the lower abdomen to fill the lungs to capacity. Then exhale slowly through the nose. Do this from 50 to 80 times and never less than 12 or 13 times. This practice oxygenates the blood, cures insomnia, removes hunger and thirst, counteracts indolence and inertia, and makes the body cooler and more comfortable. It increases the beauty and vigor of the body and helps cure disorders of the lungs. By breathing this moistened air the body becomes free from all disease. Sitkari kumbhaka enables the yogi to become cool and calm. By regularly breathing air moistened by the glands of the throat one is said to develop poetic genius and to acquire the powers of clairvoyance and clairaudience.

SITALI

Sitali is another pranayama practice in which one inhales through the mouth and exhales through the nostrils, and this exercise also helps keep the body cool. The process of sitali is similar to sitkari; either method may be used without kumbhaka when one only desires to add moisture to his system.

Turning back the tongue so that its tip is on the soft palate, inhale through the combined pressure of the tongue and the soft palate. This is called *manduka mudra*, the frog mudra, after its resemblance to a frog. Suspend the breath, and then exhale slowly through both nostrils while relaxing the whole system. This form of kumbhaka imitates a snake and makes the aspirant cool and calm. While doing this exercise one's diet should consist of milk and fruit. This kumbhaka promotes a love of study and solitude and gives one the ability to go into a trance. When one has perfected this pranayama, practicing it for one month will allow him to overcome the effects of injury. Like crabs, lobsters, serpents, lizards, frogs, salamanders, and turtles, he will be free from inflammation or fever. Through a practice like sitali kumbhaka snakes shed their skin, and they produce their hissing noise by a kind of bhastrika. Inflammations of the spleen and several other organic diseases are said to be cured by this practice.

As a result of sitali one can endure being deprived of air, water, and food, and one develops the ability to renew his skin. He is also better able to endure solitude, and he experiences intense devotion. The aspirant who can combine apana with prana is indeed happy, and if he can breathe pure air by firmly fixing his tongue against his palate, he frees himself from all disease. By "drinking" this water-saturated air daily, he becomes free of fatigue. If the aspirant practices drawing in moist air for even a short time each day there is no doubt that he will free himself from the infirmities of aging and will attain longevity.

KAKI MUDRA

In *kaki mudra* the tongue is rolled lengthwise into a trough and is protruded a little beyond the lips. Air is drawn in very slowly to fill the lungs as deeply and fully as possible. Performing the act of swallowing, one then does kumbhaka for a short time with pressure as low in the body as possible, followed by exhaling slowly through both nostrils. This practice frees one from indigestion, colic, an enlarged spleen, fever, and disorders of bile and phlegm. It is also said to cure lung troubles and counteract poison, hunger, and thirst, and it gives the practitioner a unique feeling of bliss. Drinking in the air in this manner is called kaki mudra, the crow bill mudra, after the manner of a crow, which lives a very healthy and long life. Doing this practice at dawn and twilight while visualizing the breath going to the mouth of kundalini will help the practitioner to acquire intuitive knowledge of the minds of others, an insight into the nature of objects, and knowledge of the deeper stream of life.

BHASTRIKA

This pranayama practice preserves an even temperature in the body. It is a practice similar to kapalabhati with a period of kumbhaka added. Bhastrika may be practiced in any steady, meditative asana. To perform bhastrika, inhale slowly until the abdomen is fully expanded. Then exhale forcibly through the nostrils, followed by rapid inhalation and exhalation, with the emphasis upon exhalation, making a noise that may be felt in the throat, chest, and head.

In the beginning do this 20 times or until you are fatigued. Then inhale through the right nostril, filling the abdomen. Suspend the breath and fix the gaze upon the tip of the nose, doing kumbhaka for as long as you can comfortably. Following suspension, exhale through the left nostril and inhale through the same nostril. Then again suspend the breath and exhale through the right nostril.

During bhastrika each expulsion of the breath must be sudden, and followed by an automatic inhalation, which is slower in motion. The entire process imitates the operation of a blacksmith's bellows. The exercise should be practiced slowly at the start, increasing the number of rechakas until one can do 120 exhalations a minute. Start with 10 rounds and increase to your capacity. Mula bandha may be added to this practice.

The brain has two distinct movements which are synchronous with respiration and the pulsation of the heart and its vessels. The brain increases in volume with each expiration and decreases with each inspiration, so that its volume is constantly rising and falling. This motion is also closely connected with the heart rate. If either the respiratory rate or the heart rate is accelerated, the circulation in the brain must also be increased. This brings a fresh and generous supply of blood to the brain. In bhastrika the rapid respiration accelerates the flow of the arterial blood. Whenever the circulation of the blood through the lungs is obstructed, the brain swells. At the moment of a strong exhalation the thoracic and abdominal organs are compressed, including the abdominal aorta, and more particularly the ascending branches of the aorta. Therefore more blood arrives in the head and necessarily more blood must return through the veins toward the heart. The expiration also causes an increased pressure to be exerted upon the thoracic organs, which causes a reflux of blood in the veins back toward the head. The returning arterial blood and the refluxing thoracic blood soon meet, causing the vessels to distend and blood flow to stop. This increases the pressure in the brain and the brain volume.

This phenomenon also takes place in other organs with modifications. When one inhales, blood from the vena cava and other veins is literally sucked into the chest. The jugular veins in the neck will be emptied and collapse. This decreases pressure in the brain and decreases brain volume. On the other hand, with expiration the blood is forced back into the vena cava. The more marked the respiratory movements, the more marked the effect upon the brain. Similarly, when the auricles of the heart contract, blood is again refluxed to the head. When the auricles relax, the jugular veins tend to collapse. This change is less pronounced but much more frequent than the changes with respiration. These events are additive and lead to a very irregular "beating" of the jugular vein, particularly in individuals with disease.

As a result of the practice of bhastrika the increased blood circulation throughout the body tones the nerves and furnishes them with rich red blood. This enriched and increased blood circulation adds vitality to the nerves in every part of the body by giving them a sort of massage. A prolonged practice of bhastrika energizes every atom of the body. It sets the entire system in motion and totally purifies it, thus awakening higher powers and making the aspirant a new and infinitely more powerful being.

At first body heat is augmented by the quickened circulation. This is followed by a reduction in body temperature due to profuse perspiration. When rapid blood circulation is accompanied by free perspiration, impure matter is eliminated and the strength and nourishment of the body are better maintained. The mind and body are thus able to perform their functions with greater alacrity.

Bhastrika should be practiced at least twice a day until significant heat is developed, or until the blood goes to the head and one feels pressure at the temples. At that point one should rest awhile and then continue again. When fatigue is experienced during practice, fill the lungs by inhaling through the right nostril and suspend for as long as comfortable. Then exhale slowly through the left nostril. The nose should be held tightly, without excessive pressure.

This practice corrects imbalances of vata, pitta, or kapha and increases the digestive fire, making the blood richer in quality. It increases the heart rate and the entire blood flow. It gives one great resistance to contagion or infection and may be used to prevent fever if one lives near damp and swampy places. These latter effects last for some months.

Bhastrika kumbhaka enables the yogi to alter his specific gravity at will. It increases the appetite, and is said to cure pulmonary and hepatic diseases, purify the system, destroy impurities accumulated at the entrance of brahma nadi, quickly awaken kundalini, and give great joy to those who practice it. If practiced 10 or 20 times, and followed with kumbhaka each time, it will help those suffering from impotence. It gives a sort of electric shock to the whole system. It is the finest exercise for the vascular and nervous systems, awakening or electrifying the nervous system dramatically. The rapid blood circulation in bhastrika and the vibration of the tissues of the whole body lead to the massage of the nervous, mechanical, and circulatory systems. To open the three superior valves of the *shakti nadi,* one should practice bhastrika kumbhaka. When compared with normal breathing, the oxygen consumption of each pranayama increases distinctly: 24.5 percent in ujjayi, 12.5 percent in kapalabhati, and 18.5 percent in bhastrika.

The yogic texts say that when the aspirant can fill his entire intestinal canal with air he acquires the power to cast off his skin and alter his specific gravity at will. He can decrease his specific gravity by introducing a quantity of air into his system, and can make himself heavier by compressing the inspired air within his system. He is also said to be able to appear to become plump or lean at will and to bound over the land lightly.

Bhastrika should be performed for long periods, as it breaks the barriers at three important points: the *rudra granthi* in the pelvis in the area of the *muladhara* and *svadhishthana chakras;* the *vishnu granthi* at the navel, in the *manipura chakra;* and the *brahma granthi* at the *ajna chakra* between the eyes (in some scriptures the position of these granthis varies).

Through strenuous effort all these points are made to function freely. Having awakened kundalini, bhastrika should be practiced extensively to move it upward. One may then practice other kumbhakas or not, as one desires.

Bhastrika and ujjayi are considered to be superior pranayama exercises. They should always be preceded by complete evacuation and a bath if possible. When practicing bhastrika, use ghee (clarified butter) sparingly, although buttermilk is allowed. Make the noon meal the main one.

Due to this type of respiration, chameleons can assume the appearance of plumpness or leanness. A chameleon becomes plump by inflating its lungs and intestinal canal with inspired air, and then with a single expiration it becomes lean. The long, continued hissing sound produced by serpents to alarm their prey is also due to the expulsion of a great volume of air through the nostrils. This air is taken into the lungs and intestinal canal by long and continued inspiration.

The rule is to inhale more air than necessary to oxygenate the blood, doing the deepest possible rechaka and puraka. Taking in more air than is necessary is characteristic of all hibernating animals. Through this form of kumbhaka, reptiles lighten their bodies and swim in lakes and rivers, and it enables some animals to perform bounding motions on dry land.

Surya bhedana and ujjayi produce heat; sitkari and sitali are cooling; and bhastrika preserves normal temperature. Surya bhedana destroys excess vata; ujjayi destroys excess kapha; sitkari and sitali destroy excess pitta; bhastrika balances vata, kapha, and pitta. Sitkari and sitali are more useful in hot weather; bhastrika may be done in all seasons.

Apana, being the moon, cools the body. Prana, being the sun, heats the body. The retention of breath increases longevity and augments vigor, vitality, and the spiritual force.

SAHITA KUMBHAKA

Sahita kumbhaka is of two types: with and without mantra. To practice this exercise sit in padmasana and close the nostrils, the right one with the thumb, the left with the ring finger and little finger. Then release the two fingers and inhale as slowly as you can through the left nostril. When the lungs are filled, swallow the breath, which will compress the air and give the throat muscles better tension to hold the inspired air. Do the tongue lock, jalandhara, and suspend. Holding the air in the lungs for a definite period of time, restrain it for as long as you can without pain or suffocation. Slowly exhale through the right nostril, keeping the left one closed. Immediately follow by inhaling through the right nostril, retaining the breath, and exhaling through the left nostril in the same manner as before. This process is kept up for a given length of time, inhaling through one and exhaling through the other alternately, finishing by exhaling through the left. While doing this practice the mind is focused either on the fire center at the navel, the nectar flowing from the moon in the head, or the flow of breath through the nostril.

This mode of kumbhaka should be practiced at the four quarters of the day. If practiced daily without neglect or idleness for three or more months the nadis and the nervous system will become thoroughly purified. Once the aspirant has purified his nadis, his functional defects are destroyed and he enters the first stage of yoga practice. His body becomes harmoniously developed and emits a sweet scent. His looks become pleasing and lovely, and he has cheerfulness, great courage, enthusiasm, a handsome figure, and great strength. The practice should be continued until these signs make their appearance. The attainment of these benefits may be inferred from consequent lightness of body, strength of appetite, power of digestion, and the hearing of supernormal sounds.

The ratio of the three parts of the breath in this practice should be 1:4:2—that is, 1 second of inhalation, 4 seconds of suspension, and 2 seconds of exhalation. The period of practice is determined by the student's capacity. One may start at a ratio of 4:16:8 seconds and continue at this rate until the exercise can be performed comfortably and without strain on one's capacity. Practice four times daily for periods of 48 minutes each, always ending the practice by exhaling through the left nostril, thus establishing equilibrium.

At first it is advisable to practice puraka and rechaka alone without kumbhaka for at least a week, holding to the ratio of 1:2 (one for inhalation and two for exhalation). The first week one should start with 4 seconds, then move to 8 seconds in the second week, to 12 in the third, and so on to his fullest capacity. Never hurry the increases. The aspirant should carefully watch his own capacity and then begin the practice of advanced exercises.

One should never feel it necessary to take normal breaths between any two successive rounds. Puraka, kumbhaka, and rechaka should be adjusted with care and consideration for one's capacity. These must be regulated so that they are practiced comfortably until one has full confidence in himself, and his experience justifies reaching out to greater limits. Sincere effort and perseverance will assure success if the aspirant has a systematic routine. Then kumbhaka will certainly increase. A systematic routine is also important in the practice of asana, japa, concentration, and meditation.

Puraka nourishes the spiritual growth of the aspirant and equalizes the doshas. Kumbhaka leads to stability and increases the security of life. Rechaka removes all faults. Control over exhalation gives one control over everything in the body. The secret of control over the exhalation is the control of apana.

One should always end the practice feeling invigorated and fully refreshed. Never continue the practice to a point of fatigue; instead, there should be an exhilaration of spirit following practice. Do not expose the body to drafts or take a bath immediately following the practice. Rest for 30 minutes or so before doing anything else. Have a systematic practice and develop it to a high degree.

Without personal help and guidance from someone well practiced in this process the student should not venture beyond the ratio of 16:64:32 seconds. Sahita kumbhaka should be practiced within this ratio until the air can easily be confined within the body. If one develops his practice to this ratio and performs it with mastery he will be amply rewarded, and the necessary further guidance will come in due time.

To measure the regulation of the breath, 12 moments have been laid down. A moment, called *matra* in Sanskrit, consists of the time taken by the blink of an eyelid, a single clap of the hands, or the utterance of a short letter. Nowadays the time value is usually set by simply counting slowly the number of seconds chosen for the ratio, or one may use the mantra given him by his guru.

Another process is to do pranayama as given above, with the addition of an external kumbhaka. On exhaling, the breath is made to remain outside the lungs for some 10 to 20 seconds. The exercise may be done according to this pattern: inhale 5 or 10 seconds, suspend for 10 to 20 seconds, exhale 5 to 10 seconds, and then suspend externally 10 to 20 seconds. Then proceed as before. These practices give the aspirant control over the nerve centers and prana.

The best pranayama ratio is 20:80:40 seconds. An average ratio is 16:64:32, and the lowest is 12:48:24. One should prolong the process of kumbhaka gradually; carefully note the various mental and physical changes going on in the system while practicing.

THREE STAGES OF PRACTICE

In the first stage of this practice the student will find that the exercise induces a considerable amount of perspiration. Practice should be done until perspiration appears at the eyebrows, armpits, nose, and the joints. This purifies the body and is known as *adhama pranayama*. Until the body is purified this perspiration should be removed with a towel because it contains many impurities. After the body becomes purified the perspiration should be massaged back into the body to make it strong. At this stage if one experiences a sense of suffocation he need not be concerned, for it will soon pass.

The second stage brings the body to a place where one may feel a quivering sensation, unconscious muscular reflexes, tremors of the face or other parts, or even a vibration of the whole body. This will gradually taper off and be replaced by a peculiar sensation of motion along the spinal cord, like the leaping of a frog. As the practice becomes more perfect, this peculiar leaping sensation will cease. This may be a physical sensation, or it may result in the actual movement of the body. This is called *madhyama pranayama*.

The highest practice, *uttama pranayama*, is said to bring the practitioner to the point where he may suspend himself in the air by merely resting the toes or fingertips on the ground. It is said that in time he will find himself able to bound about like an inflated rubber balloon. The texts indicate that special practices will enable him to walk on water and to perform similar feats. Such an accomplished yogi does not want to be known to others. He may then live in such a manner that others think he is out of his mind. This sort of deception is consciously created by certain adepts so that they are not disturbed.

One school of spiritual seekers practices by first inhaling and exhaling in such a subtle way that one cannot even hear the breath; then, following an inhalation, suspending the breath and counting to 120. They then exhale in the same manner as the inhalation. This count is gradually increased, and one's aim is to be able to suspend a feather before the nose and mouth and to exhale so sparingly that the feather will not move or stir at all. In this practice one abstains from legumes and from the grains of rice, millet, and corn. Training is also provided in which one embraces a number of mental and moral conditions. One must have a comprehensive knowledge of the meaning of life and constantly be aware of his goal. He must practice non-attachment, which will help free him from sensual desire and produce a temperament of kindness and benevolence.

With regular practice one can control prana in six months. Then vayu enters the middle channel, sushumna. Then the aspirant can conquer his roving mind, restrain his breath and sexual energy, and obtain success in all walks of life.

MAHA VEDHA

Maha vedha is an advanced practice whereby prana is forced to leave its normal course through ida and pingala and enter sushumna. Prior to the practice of maha vedha, other advanced practices, such as *maha mudra* and *maha bandha,* are perfected. Maha mudra and maha bandha are useless without performing maha vedha. One must practice these three alternately. If possible, practice them four times daily. Perfecting maha vedha allows the aspirant to gain control of the breath, and enables him to penetrate sushumna and the brahma nadi. By doing this, the old may regain their youthfulness and become free from all diseases. To perform maha vedha, the lungs are filled completely. Combining the vayus of *prana, apana,* and *samana,* gently and evenly press the sides of the upper abdomen. The hands are placed beside the body and it is raised off the floor slightly. Then the body is dropped, striking the buttocks on the floor gently, causing prana to leave ida and pingala and go to sushumna. This is practiced only by accomplished yogis.

AN ADVANCED TECHNIQUE IN PRANAYAMA

There are a great many methods of pranayama. Some practitioners stress one technique, and some another. For the most part these methods produce their results very slowly, and some techniques are of little use whatsoever. The following technique is known only to those advanced yogis who are accomplished and who are satisfied with nothing less than the shortest and most heroic means of attaining their goal.

This technique should be followed only under the direct guidance and supervision of a master. Those who have not completed the necessary preparations either will be wasting their time or may actually bring about significant harm to themselves. Before attempting this practice one should be experienced in the basic pranayama exercises as well as in the basic methods of purification, including *neti, dhauti,* and *basti.* One should also have perfected his asana and the necessary mudras. For those who are accomplished in those practices this pranayama technique will yield excellent results.

To begin the practice drink about four mouthfuls of cool, fresh water, and then sit in siddhasana or padmasana. Make sure that the head, neck, and trunk are in a straight line, and close the mouth, keeping the teeth firmly pressed together. Close the eyes gently, focus the attention on the bridge of the nose, and then observe the breathing. Exhale all the breath from the lungs. To make sure that every possible vestige of air is eliminated from the lungs, make three final exclamations of "uh," a sort of grunt. Place the thumb of the right hand on the right nostril, the ring finger and little finger on the left nostril, and close the right nostril. Inhale to your capacity through the left nostril. When the lungs are filled, swallow as if to swallow saliva, drop the chin into the neck (jalandhara), and retain the breath. The hand may now be returned to the knees or kept in position. Count slowly to 50 or to your own capacity. You should not hold the breath beyond your capacity or to the point of forcing yourself to gasp.

When you have reached that limit, close the left nostril and allow the air to escape slowly through the right nostril to a distance of four inches, or until the tension in the lungs has been reduced somewhat. (The mind can be trained to measure the subtleties of breath and cannot be mistaken in the advanced stages. When the aspirant practices pranayama for a considerable length of time the length of breath comes under his control.) Then inhale through the right nostril, filling the lungs again. Immediately after that let the same quantity of air slowly pass out of the left nostril, and then take it in again as before. Then alternate to the right nostril and complete the same process. This process of short breathing should be continued until the capacity to retain the breath becomes exhausted. Then empty the lungs slowly until every vestige of air is eliminated, and resume normal respiration.

Rest for a period before resuming the technique. While resting, keep the mind empty and do not allow it any action; establish only *unmani*—a state in which conscious thoughts are not allowed to function. The teeth should be kept firmly pressed together during the entire round of practice. In one round of this pranayama, the lungs are filled and the surface tension in the lungs is reduced a little, and is then again reestablished by a process of short breathing. This process is continued until one's capacity to retain the breath any longer has been exhausted. Then the lungs are finally emptied completely.

In the beginning, the breath will naturally tend to escape more completely on each short breath, but this must be controlled in the manner described. Never allow the breath to escape quickly from the lungs or permit them to empty completely at any time.

After the rest period repeat the process; this time begin by inhaling with the right nostril. Continue with the practice of alternating from one nostril to the other with each complete pranayama as well as during the short breathing process. After some practice this short breathing may be continued for about five minutes. At the completion of each round sit quietly with the hands resting on the knees or thighs, make the mind empty, and fix the attention between the eyebrows.

After having developed this practice, the second round should be altered in this manner: empty the lungs completely and end the first round with a rest period. Begin at once to fill the lungs, through the right nostril, allowing only four inches of air to enter at this nostril. Then shift to the left and inhale, and then again to the right. Continue until the lungs are completely filled. The last inhalation should be taken in through the right nostril. When the swallowing technique is done, retain to the same count as before, and then start the short breathing until the power to sustain the breath is exhausted. Next the lungs are slowly and completely emptied by uttering the sound "uh" and pressing the abdomen in with each sound.

In this process of short breathing, only the surface tension should be allowed to escape. The air should be allowed to flow down only about four inches from the nostrils. Naturally the entire quantity of air will want to rush out, but it is important that one prevent this from happening. The inhalation and exhalation must be done slowly. Kumbhaka should be done only to one's capacity and never to an extreme. One should increase the length of the suspension slowly over many practice sessions. One should remember that he is dealing with a power that must be developed gradually.

Diet must be considered from the standpoint of the individual and his physical condition. An adequate amount of milk and ghee (clarified butter) should always be consumed. Ghee must be taken cautiously at the start according to one's power of digestion and assimilation. Three meals a day may be taken initially if one fills his stomach only to one-fourth of its capacity at the morning meal, three-fourths at the midday meal, and only half a stomachful in the evening. Black pepper and ginger may be taken to aid in digestion and to warm the stomach. Something sour may be taken to flavor the food as needed. Barley, wheat, rice, green gram (fresh chana, not dried), ghee, and milk are the staple articles of food. Pure cane sugar may be used for sweetening. As one develops this practice the diet must be further simplified and should eventually consist almost entirely of liquids. However, this cannot and should not be done at the start, as it will lead to disastrous results. Approximately 30 minutes should elapse after a practice before food is eaten, but a small glass of milk may be taken immediately.

In this technique of pranayama the air will eventually begin to enter the esophagus and stomach in small quantities and will finally reach the bowels. At this point some pain will be felt, and the practitioner must endure a reasonable amount of it. The practice will progress slowly until all pain disappears and the stomach and bowels can be freely filled with air.

When one has control of kumbhaka the experience of hunger lessens, and one may live on only milk and a few sweet fruits. One develops the ability to float easily on water, and his physical powers increase remarkably. At that point one can begin to practice concentration of the mind. With regard to sexual practices, one may indulge a few times per month with no detriment but must be cautious and conserve his vital fluid to the utmost.

If one seeks to master the breath in a hurry, he will fail. It is only when one has gained more and more experience with the slow development of his capacity that he can develop the powers that accrue from the regular practice of pranayama.

The student may begin by practicing three times a day: morning, noon, and evening. At each sitting he may do as many rounds of pranayama as possible without exhausting his energy; one should never rise from his seat tired or worn from his practice. If one does this practice steadily, slowly, and patiently every day without a break, he will observe positive results. In time the breath will be found to create less tension in the body and will be easier to restrain; it will then flow comfortably throughout the body.

At first one may notice that at the completion of the practice the nerves are tense and slight tremors may occur. There is no need for anxiety about this if one consumes enough wheat, barley, rich milk, and ghee with his meals. In time this will pass. In the beginning one will also perspire freely. This perspiration must not be wiped off but should instead be massaged into the body as if it were an oil bath.

Fifty counts or seconds of kumbhaka is sufficient at the start, and one should stay at this level for at least two months. When this can be easily done, the period may be increased to 75 seconds. If pain develops it will pass in the course of two months or earlier. Only when the pain has subsided should one further lengthen the retention period.

When one has reached 100 seconds of kumbhaka he should exhale to the navel, and then inhale this same amount immediately and repeat kumbhaka for another 100 seconds. Then, exhaling through the opposite nostril to the distance of the navel, one should immediately inhale and repeat the kumbhaka for another 100 counts. This should be repeated until he has done kumbhaka from one to five times. Then one may lengthen the kumbhaka to 125 seconds, breathing alternately through the left nostril, then through the right nostril, and finally through both nostrils. Slowly one may increase kumbhaka to 150 or 200 seconds or more, according to his capacity. The longer the period of kumbhaka, the more freely the body will perspire.

Kumbhaka increases the heat in the body. To mitigate this, when the heat becomes too intense the practice may be done in water. Twice a week one may also massage the body from the top of the head to the feet with a special mixture. This mixture is composed of almond milk, almond oil, black pepper or ginger juice, saffron, and other ingredients that are cooling by nature. This mixture may be applied and left on for half an hour or more to allow it to soak in.

When the full kumbhaka attempted is completed, one should allow the breath to escape in small gusts or bursts alternately through first one nostril and then the other until the lungs are deflated. Then one should inhale and perform kumbhaka as outlined above, doing the short breath to the navel after each kumbhaka. This process should be followed in the three formats described earlier, creating the equivalent of 3 x 400, or 1,200 seconds of suspension. Gradually one may increase this process until he attains the level of 3,000 to 5,000 seconds of suspension.

At this point one is able to detect air beginning to enter the alimentary canal. The air will tend to remain in the lungs until about 4,000 seconds of kumbhaka are reached. After that point it will force its way out of the lungs and attempt to enter the alimentary canal, kicking back against the throat to enter the esophagus and stomach. The yogi may aid in this by swallowing and pressing the chin into the hollow of the neck, applying jalandhara. In this process the air will encounter an obstruction in its downward movement. It will again rebound to the throat and will try for a deeper entry into the esophagus if the practitioner maintains his throat lock. This process will go on in a similar manner throughout its progress into and through the entire alimentary tract. When the air reaches the anus, mula bandha must be applied to prevent its exit. Pain will develop and may initially be quite acute, but as time progresses it will disappear and the process will become quite easy and natural. During this time the bowels will croak and the air may be felt moving below the navel from one side to the other.

Before starting this practice of pranayama take about four mouthfuls of water to prepare for the air to enter the alimentary canal. At meals it will similarly be advantageous to eat a small amount of barley, wheat, or rice, well soaked with ghee to lubricate and facilitate the entry of food into the stomach and bowels. The greater one's capacity for kumbhaka, the longer he will be free from hunger. This is the result of air circulating throughout the alimentary canal and is referred to by the yogis as "living on air." When one attains this stage he should consume only rich milk and a little sweet fruit. He may then seriously begin the practice of concentration and meditation.

Pranayama may be considered to be properly developed when kumbhaka can be done for some 5 or 6 minutes. At this stage the yogi may begin training the mind for one-pointedness. The mind will soon become absorbed wherever the attention is directed. When this occurs the aspirant may then undertake the awakening of kundalini. However, if the mind becomes restless because of these strenuous pranayama and meditation exercises, then one should learn to relax.

With regard to diet, one should initially observe a strict diet of green gram, which is ground, fried, and mixed with the same quantity of boiled barley, wheat, or rice, ghee, and a pinch of salt. This may be eaten once a day at the noon hour. This diet will facilitate the entry of the air into the alimentary canal. After this takes place the diet must be changed and limited to the more liquid foods, such as barley broth. The quantity of solid food consumed amounts to about 21 tablespoonfuls, which must be reduced at the ratio of a tablespoonful a day for nine days. Then unleavened bread of wheat or barley, and ghee, milk, and a little sweet fruit may be substituted. Ground whole wheat and an equal quantity of vegetables may be boiled together and eaten with curds well sprinkled with ginger, cumin seed, and other spices, as well as a small amount of salt. To reduce the extra heat developed by the practice of kumbhaka, spices should be fried in ghee and then added to the food.

THE METHOD OF
THE GREATER KUMBHAKA

Close the left nostril and inhale slowly through the right. Follow that with kumbhaka to 15,000 counts. Then exhale through the right nostril and immediately inhale through the left. Repeat the kumbhaka for 15,000 counts. Continue this process until four such pranayamas are completed. Then close the right nostril and exhale through the left to a distance of four inches. Immediately inhale this same quantity of air through the same nostril, allowing the breath to play back and forth to the same distance through this same nostril. At the same time retain most of the air in the lungs and complete the practice as directed above. This practice will yield a net kumbhaka of 60,000 seconds. This unusual length of time can be maintained only by the accomplished yogi.

Next, inhale through the right and do kumbhaka to the extent of 12,000 seconds (3 hours 20 minutes). Then sit in concentration for 10 minutes. Repeat the process through the left nostril and follow with concentration. Finally repeat this through both nostrils. As a result the senses will cease their activity and one will forget himself. He will enter into a superconscious state of self-absorption, transcending the limits of relative and conditional existence, and entering into union with the universal spirit.

Gradually one should be able to control the breath for 1½ hours, at which point psychic powers will manifest themselves. When one has been able to hold his breath for 3,000 to 5,000 counts he will be able to feel it throughout the body. There will be a tingling and stinging sensation over the entire surface of the body that will disappear on exhalation. If one wishes to progress rapidly he must do kumbhaka without fear and must tolerate all of these experiences. One must watch the diet so that his digestion remains good. One should always have a sufficient amount of ghee or oily food to keep the nerves soothed and the body properly lubricated. He should begin his practice slowly and with careful patience, controlling the breath little by little. In this manner one will surely succeed.

chapter three

SVARODAYA:
THE SCIENCE OF BREATH

No science that explains life in the universe is so satisfying, grand, and complete as the science of breath. It is said in the yoga texts that the breath (prana) is the inseparable power (shakti) of the universal life force, the supreme of all created things, and the life principle of the universe. Prana is the substratum in which all causes and effects are held like beads on a thread. As spokes are held in the hub of a wheel, all things are sustained in the breath. The universal life force breathed forth or exhaled the universe, and it will, in the end, inhale the universe back into itself. In its extent and scope, prana is as incomprehensible as the ocean of infinity.

In chapter one, the word *prana* was defined as "breath." *Prana* also means "energy." The word *prana* itself comes from the Sanskrit root *pra*, meaning "first," and *na*, which means "the smallest unit of energy," so *prana* itself means "the first breath, or the most basic unit of energy." Prana is the universal force, and all action is merely a change of the phase or aspect of prana. Prana is brought into existence and kept in activity by the center of consciousness.

Prana is the life principle, the dynamic or working force in human beings and in all life forms. It is the power which is the support of the body and all its moving life forces. The nadis, the subtle energy paths of the body, are channels for prana. The body is the support for the nadis. When prana is in motion and flows through the nadis, consciousness arises. Greater consciousness, light, wisdom, and truth, which are all-pervading but latent, are awakened by regulating the motion of the *pranic* vehicles.

The science of breath has its foundation in the desire to control and understand prana. This science of breath is of the highest importance to any student of yoga, and is the most useful, comprehensive, and interesting branch of yoga. It is said in yoga texts that the wise should study the regulation of prana if they desire to suspend the activity of the mind or concentrate their will upon the achievement of yoga. Control of the breath leads to health, an increase in strength and energy, good complexion, increased vitality, the growth of knowledge, and the extension of the life span.

It is the breath and prana that maintain the constituents of the body, such as the blood, flesh, and marrow. Prana is the impetus and origin of movements of diverse kinds. It restrains the mind from undesirable objects and concentrates the mind upon objects that are desirable.

Prana causes the ten senses of perception and action to perform their appropriate functions. It bears all the sensory impressions and sensations to the mind. Prana is the force which holds together the elements of the body and assists in the very cohesion of atomic particles. It gives form to the embryo in the womb. The flow of breath and prana in the body furnishes the proof of the existence of life. Prana is the cause of speech, touch, sound, and scent, and is the origin of joy and cheerfulness. It ignites the internal fire which maintains warmth and metabolism.

Prana also expels all impurities. It penetrates all the channels of the body, both gross and fine, and disposes of all disease. Prana, through the breath, achieves all these functions when the breath is balanced and undisturbed. It is the motion of the prana in the nadis that awakens consciousness, which is all-pervading but veiled.

Prana is lost from the body in exhalation, excessive exercise, the elimination of waste, the emission of semen, the process of childbirth, and in times of great emotion. If prana is not regulated the system does not receive an adequate supply of oxygen. The absence of appetite may also indicate an imbalance in prana.

If prana recedes from any part of the body, whatever the cause, that part loses its power of action. Death is caused by the outgoing of prana; the gasps of a dying man are considered to be like a reversed breath. At death, the prana exits by way of either the eyes, ears, nose, navel, rectum, urethra, or fontanel, leaving an impression at the site of its exit. Its tendency is to leave the body from the site where the mind dwells instinctively or where the innermost feelings reside.

THE VAYUS

The universal life force, the prana, when present in human beings gives birth to the breath. On entering the human being prana divides itself into five major functions called vayus, which are prefixed with a special term according to their individual function. These are *prana vayu, apana vayu, samana vayu, udana vayu,* and *vyana vayu.*

Vayu is usually defined as air or ether, one of the five constituents of the universe. At a more subtle level, vayu is not merely air, but the medium in which air exists and the force by which it is held together. The word *vayu* comes from the root *va*, which means "motion" or "that which flows." Just as vayu is the vehicle for the manifestation of desires, inclinations, and motions, so is air the vehicle for vayu. Modern science divides air into various elements such as carbon, oxygen, hydrogen, and nitrogen. However, the practitioner of pranayama must also be aware of other subtler qualities of air, including its function, energies, and place of residence.

In the terrestrial sphere there are actually forty-nine types of vayu. The modifications of prana that reside in the body take on various names according to their functions, but all are known by the generic term *vayu*. Ten of these forty-nine are responsible for directing and administrating our mental and physical activities. Of these ten, the five named above—prana, apana, samana, vyana, and udana—are most important from a yogic point of view.

The fourteen most important nadis in the body are either weak or strong according to the amount of prana that flows through them. By controlling vayu as it moves through the nadis, an aspirant gains extraordinary force and energy. As indicated in chapter one, it is the purpose of pranayama to bring vayu under control. Until the aspirant brings vayu under control he cannot attain freedom from the snare of births and deaths; therefore the aspirant who desires liberation persists in his practices.

In the *Prana Gopana Tapani Upanishad* one reads: "Air, which is one element, becomes five on entering the world, and is so manifested in each body." The first of these functions is prana vayu, the subtle vayu that nourishes life. Prana vayu is concerned with respiration and the function of the heart. The more prana the body takes in, the stronger and longer is one's life. The second is apana vayu, which acts to eliminate waste matter from the system, as in urination, defecation, gestation, and ejaculation. The third is samana vayu, and its purpose is to separate the food nutrients from the waste elements. The fourth, udana vayu, is upward-running, involved with speech, and with forcing air out of the lungs. The fifth, vyana vayu, helps supply energy to the senses and the blood and deals with the entire body. It coordinates all the pranic vehicles and allows for the general motion of the body. Among these functions, prana vayu and apana vayu are the most significant, because they perform the foremost work in the body.

PRANA VAYU

Prana vayu governs the region between the larynx and the base of the heart. Its specific locus, or seat, is the heart. Its energy has an upward motion, and thus it is sometimes called the ascending air. To take anything into oneself requires the work of prana, and so the processes of inhalation, of swallowing, and even of opening one's mouth are the result of the power of prana. Prana also involves the process of taking in sensory impressions, so prana affects the organs located at the eyes, ears, nose, and tongue.

Prana vayu is described as having the color of a blood-red gem. The prana within gathers at the navel and from there it is distributed throughout the whole body. It functions with great power in the head, especially at the tip of the nostrils, but its strength is also reflected throughout the body, down to one's toes.

The energy of prana is utilized in the assimilation of food during digestion, and in the action of the vital organs, especially the heart. It also works to maintain a proper temperature for the body in response to extremes of heat or cold. On the mental side, it involves the processes of taking in information, assimilating, and integrating it.

APANA VAYU

Apana vayu has its primary influence below the navel, and its seat or primary abode is said to be in the rectum. Apana is the aspect of the life force which involves the ability to throw off, eliminate, and eject what is not needed or useful to the system. Apana governs the functions of the kidneys, colon, rectum, bladder, and genitals. It circulates from the navel to the toes, although it moves primarily in the rectum. The better and more efficient one's elimination processes, the better the control of the apana vayu. When apana and prana are both purified, the quantities of urine and excrement decrease. When apana is not functioning properly there is poor elimination of all wastes; exhalation may not efficiently eliminate waste gases, and hence the blood may be unable to receive adequate oxygen. On the mental side, disorders of apana tend to slow one down. When apana is not regulated one lacks motivation or inclination. He feels lazy, sluggish, heavy, dull, and mentally befuddled.

SAMANA VAYU

Samana governs the region between the heart and the navel, and regulates all the metabolic activity involved in digestion. Its specific seat is said to be the navel and intestines, and it affects the pancreas, liver, and stomach. Its work is to digest the food and separate the nutrients from waste.

When samana vayu is in disorder a person may eat well and have a good appetite, yet be unable to properly assimilate food. When this happens the nutritive and waste elements in food are not properly separated and the body may retain toxins. Then the breath becomes short and one may develop a gastric disorder. This may occur in those who fast excessively and then abruptly begin to eat, or in those who are convalescing.

On the mental level, samana separates desirable from undesirable thoughts and gives one the power of discrimination. When it is imbalanced one may be delirious, delusional, or unsound of mind. Samana vayu is also considered to be an organizing force.

UDANA VAYU

Udana is the opposite of prana in its function. It forces air out of the lungs and body, and is concerned with speech and the production of sound. Udana rules the body above the larynx and is located in the throat.

When udana is unregulated, speech is uncoordinated and one cannot speak properly. Imbalances in udana may also cause shortness of breath or other respiratory irregularities. It also causes the voice to break or crack and prevents one from developing a sense of pitch. Vomiting is also governed by udana, and imbalances in this vayu may produce the desire to vomit.

VYANA VAYU

Vyana pervades the entire body and is a coordinating, connecting force in the body. It has no specific locus or seat. Its function is to connect and coordinate all the other powers, such as the ability to have sensory awareness throughout the body. It controls the cutaneous system (the skin), and thus goose bumps and perspiration are experienced because of it. Vyana vayu also governs the senses of touch, taste, sight, and hearing. Because of vyana one can coordinate the body's movements and move all its parts through nerve impulses. Vyana also controls the muscular system and governs the relaxation and contraction of all muscles, both voluntary and involuntary. Vyana coordinates balance, regulates the cerebrospinal system, and generally deals with the way we react to and interact with our environment.

When vyana is imbalanced there is a lack of coordination and balance in the body. In such a condition the coordination between body and mind is also lost: on the mental level the thought process is inconsistent and the thoughts are ever changing. Derangements in vyana may also involve disruptions in the ability of the body to perceive sensations.

The yoga texts also describe other supplementary vayus. *Naga vayu* performs the function of belching and produces clarity of mind. *Kurma vayu* governs expansion and contraction, such as the opening and closing of the eyelids; it is also connected to the sensory nerves. *Krikara vayu* induces hunger and thirst, and causes sneezing. *Devadatta vayu*, responsible for yawning, like vyana, pervades the whole body. It remains with the body for some time after death. *Dhananjaya vayu* governs the ability to hiccough. These last five vayus operate on a physical plane only and regulate the physiological functions of the material body; they are not given special emphasis or consideration in yogic training. One additional vayu that is mentioned is *maha vayu*, which is related to the functioning of the brain.

Pranayama is the means of controlling the vayus, the five divisions or vehicles of the breath. Therefore the wise should study the regulation of prana if they desire to suspend the dissipated activity of the mind and concentrate their will upon the goal of yoga, self-enlightenment.

THE SOLAR AND LUNAR BREATHS AND THEIR RELATIONSHIP TO THE TATTVAS

The *Svarodaya Vivarana* is an esoteric tantric text which deals with the science of breath and the tattvas. It is highly complex and its advanced knowledge is not comprehended by most students; only one who has perfected pranayama practice can make use of the knowledge it contains. The whole aim of this text is to explain the qualities and attributes of the tattvas and to describe how and why they are used. A small part of that complex body of knowledge is provided here, to encourage the study of the tattvas as the student becomes competent on the path of yoga.

Much of the system of the science of breath is written in language that is poetic and metaphorical, and which is understood by only a fortunate few. For example, the texts say that the moon falls from heaven, giving the nectar of life to the lotuses (plexuses) that arise in the body. The texts further state that, by the constant practice of right action and yoga science, one becomes immortal by imbibing the "lunar nectar." The lamps of the tattvas also are said to receive their oil from the moon. The aspirant is encouraged to protect it from the solar force so that longevity is increased. A competent teacher is able to explain the profound knowledge hidden within these symbolic expressions to the prepared aspirant.

When one succeeds in regulating the breath he will be able to understand all the various aspects and phases of the breath. This is the special art of svarodaya, the science of the tattvas. Just as there are some aspirants who practice only hatha yoga, so also are there some who devote themselves and their entire energies to the study and practice of svarodaya.

One basic distinction in the science of svarodaya is that of the solar and lunar breaths. The breath which flows in the right nostril is described as hot, and that flowing in the left as cold. Thus the right nadi is called the sun or solar breath (pingala) and the left nadi is known as the moon or lunar breath (ida). The energy which flows in the right nostril produces heat in the body. It is stimulating and conducts energy toward the organs of the body; it promotes digestion and strength. The energy in the left nadi has a cooling effect and is inhibitory to the organs.

Although most people believe that they generally breathe through both nostrils, the ancient texts of svarodaya and modern science together confirm that the breath alternates between the two nostrils. This results in one nostril being dominant at any point in time. When this action is normal, nostril dominance will alternate approximately every 1 hour 50 minutes. These rhythms are perfectly tuned only in one who is practiced in pranayama.

In the average person the alternations in the dominance of the left and right nostrils in breathing vary greatly due to both subtle and gross causes within the individual. For example, disease, habits, and food intake all have an influence on the breath and may divert it from its normal flow. If the breath in one nostril continues to be dominant for a longer period than 1 hour 50 minutes it clearly indicates imbalance. This may be due to an excess of heat or cold. The function of the alternation of the nostrils in breathing is to maintain an equilibrium in the body temperature.

A person in good health begins to breathe through ida, the left nostril, at sunrise, or about six o'clock, on the first day following the new moon. As already stated, the breath continues its flow through this same nostril for about 1 hour 50 minutes. Then the dominant flow changes to the right nostril, and continues to alternate back and forth about every two hours throughout the whole twenty-four hours.

The same pattern will be followed for the next two days, making a total of three days. Then at sunrise on the fourth day the breath will begin in the right nostril, pingala, and continue to alternate in the manner described for three days. Every three days this pattern will alternate. On the first day of the dark fortnight, the day of the full moon, the right breath, pingala, will begin to flow at sunrise and the same order of changes will go on during this half phase of the moon.

The breathing pattern changes in every sign of the zodiac. This means that the dominant breath becomes either the solar or lunar breath in accordance with the sign into which the moon enters. The moon takes approximately twenty-eight days to complete its course. The first fourteen days of this period are the bright fortnight of the waxing moon, and the next fourteen are the dark fortnight of the waning moon. During these two fortnights the moon travels through all twelve signs of the zodiac, remaining in each sign about sixty hours. The breath makes thirty-one changes during this time. Each fortnight is subdivided into five parts of about three days each, and each day of twenty-four hours is subdivided into twelve parts of two hours each.

In the bright fortnight of the waxing moon the left breath is more powerful, and in the dark fortnight, during the waning moon, the right breath is more powerful. During the daytime the solar breath passes through Aries, Gemini, Leo, Libra, Sagittarius, and Aquarius, at which positions the breath changes to pingala. During the night the lunar breath passes through Taurus, Cancer, Virgo, Scorpio, Capricorn, and Pisces, positions at which the breath changes to ida. This natural process should be reversed by the aspirant, making ida, the lunar breath, flow in the daytime, and pingala, the solar breath, flow at night.

The sun has six months of a southern circuit and six months of a northern circuit. When the sun is in Capricorn the northern circuit begins; it ends when the

sun is in Gemini. When the sun is in Cancer the southern
circuit begins; it ends when the sun is in Sagittarius. These
twelve months are divided into six parts of two months
each, each two months representing one season in the traditional Indian system. The sun passes through Pisces and
Aries in spring, through Taurus and Gemini in summer,
through Cancer and Leo in the rainy season, through
Virgo and Libra in fall, through Scorpio and Sagittarius in
what is traditionally called the midseason, and through
Capricorn and Aquarius in the winter. In the northern circuit are spring, summer, and the rainy season. In the
southern circuit are fall, winter, and the midseason.

The breath also has its seasons in the circuit of the day.
Morning corresponds to spring, noontime to summer, and
the afternoon to the rainy season. The evening corresponds to fall, midnight to winter, and the last part of the
night to the midseason.

For a *svara yogi* the breath begins to flow in its dominant
nostril just before sunrise and continues to make its orderly
changes during the day. In the bright fortnight the left
breath begins first. This lunar breath will be especially
powerful on Monday, Wednesday, Thursday, and Friday.
On the dark fortnight the right breath will become active
at sunrise and will be more powerful on Tuesday, Saturday,
and Sunday. On Thursday of the waxing moon, ida will
flow first. On Thursday of the waning moon, pingala will
flow first. On Saturday at the beginning of both day and
night, pingala will flow first. By observing these patterns
and doing only acts that are suitable to the flow of either
ida or pingala (whichever is dominant at the time), the yogi
has success in all his acts.

The body is a miniature counterpart of the whole universe. As the sun and the moon constantly move in their
northern and southern orbits in the macrocosm, they are

also traveling in the microcosm of the body, through the influence of ida and pingala during both day and night. The moon travels by the left nadi, ida, and bedews the whole system with nectar. The sun travels by the right nadi, pingala, and dries the system moistened by the nectar. When the sun and moon meet at the muladhara chakra, that is called *amavashya,* the new moon day. Close by, *kundalini* sleeps in *adharakunda.* The aspirant who wishes to rouse kundalini seeks to control his mind and to confine the moon to its place and the sun to its place, so that the moon cannot shed its nectar nor can the sun dry it. When this occurs and when at the same time the place of nectar becomes dried by the *svadhishthana* fire with the help of vayu, then kundalini awakens herself.

The alternation of the breath is brought about by the mucous membranes in the nostrils, which become hot, swollen, and in a state of erection on the side in which the breath is not flowing freely. The nadi produces this condition and causes the breath to change from one nostril to the other. In this process the breath goes through five changes. At one point it reaches to approximately the navel, 16 finger-widths from the nose. At a later point it reaches to the end of the sternum, about 12 finger-widths. Later, at a third point, it terminates about 8 finger-widths from the nose, at the middle of the sternum. Next the breath terminates at the chin, about 4 finger-widths from the nose. Finally, when it is running in the heart chakra it terminates just above the upper lip, and is scarcely felt coming out of the nostril at all. After the left nostril passes through these changes, then the right does likewise.

One may also observe another cycle: for the first 15 minutes the breath flows out of the lower part of the nostril, during the second 15 minutes it flows out of the forward part of the nostril, and for the third 15 minutes it flows out both of the nostrils. These changes take place while the breath is flowing through ida and pingala as just described.

When the body is functioning perfectly, the students of the science of svarodaya are able to calculate the exact time of day and determine the nature of events by the rhythmic erectility of the nasal mucous membrane, because its alternating engorgement is so clocklike in regularity. This alternating erectility of the mucous membrane also enables one to study the function of the sympathetic nervous system and the mechanism which regulates the heart.

If the left armpit is pressed by lying on the left side or by other means, the right nostril will permit air to flow freely through it. If the right armpit is pressed, the left nostril flows freely. If an individual's left nostril cavity is blocked by a physical disorder, such as polypoid growths, nasal-pharyngeal adenoids, a deviated septum, or other ailments, the person is likely to suffer from biliousness or tachycardia. When a stenosis from a similar obstruction occurs on the right side, the individual may suffer from repeated catarrhal inflammations of various mucous membranes.

From midnight until noon, prana flows in the nerves; this means that the energy in the nerves is most active at that time. From noon until midnight, prana flows in the blood vessels; thus its effect is greater on these vessels during this period. At noon and at midnight, the energy becomes equal in both systems of nadis. At sunset, prana has passed into the blood vessels in full strength, and at dawn, prana is passing into the spine, which is the course of the sun, the solar current of prana.

When one is in perfect health there is an even exchange of prana in the nadis, and the positive and negative currents flow in regular order and in definite channels. The force of free will, as well as certain other forces, may change the nature of the local prana and affect the negative and positive flow to various degrees. The character of the flow of pranic energy is the truest indication and most perfect record of the tattvic changes in the body: when these currents are balanced one reflects health, and their imbalance indicates disease. Thus the aspirant should bring these currents into balance. On the first lunar day one should make the lunar breath, ida, flow during the whole day, and the solar breath, pingala, during the whole night. One should always act in accord with the dominance of ida or pingala. For example, the aspirant should eat solids only when the air flows freely through the right nostril. At night, when it flows freely through the left nadi, he should rest. To those who practice keeping the sun and moon in their proper order the knowledge of the past and future becomes easy and clear. He who practices this is truly a yogi.

When the breath remains dominant in either nostril for over twenty-four hours, it clearly indicates the presence of some illness. If this lasts a longer time it means a serious illness, and when one nostril dominates for two or three days, then one is due to become extremely ill. If the breath goes to the fire center, the navel, for some time, it indicates that the nerve currents going to that center are excessive. If the breath remains there for a longer period than normal, it means that those ganglia are overworked. A similar pattern exists with the other nerve centers, or chakras.

THE TATTVAS

There are five important chakras—*muladhara, svadhishthana, manipura, anahata,* and *vishuddha*—which correspond respectively to the constituents of earth *(prithivi),* water *(apas),* fire *(tejas* or *agni),* air *(vayu),* and ether *(akasha).* Each chakra is the vehicle or carrier of a unique and distinct form of consciousness. Each of the five centers influences the breath, depending upon the body habits and activities, which may cause these centers to work either insufficiently or overtime. The center through which the breath passes forces its own momentum and energy through the nerve currents. It is these nerve currents that direct the breath to flow an average of approximately a thousand times an hour.

Each of these currents influences the constituent of the body corresponding to the center active at the time: for example, if the breath is in the water center, the fluids of the body are being influenced. The exercises and practices of yoga are done with the aim of freeing the movement of prana in these centers, and thus developing the chakras to reveal the powers that lie hidden there. As indicated in the accompanying table, each chakra has a given number of important nadis or nerve currents that are symbolized by lotus petals (and that, apart from their physical duties, also have a definite metaphysical meaning); the order and amount of time in which, in a truly healthy person, the breath normally remains in each center while flowing through ida or pingala is also indicated.

Chakra	Tattva	Petals	Minutes
muladhara	earth (prithivi)	4	20
svadhishthana	water (apas)	6	16
manipura	fire (tejas)	10	12
anahata	air (vayu)	12	8
vishuddha	ether (akasha)	16	4

The force of prithivi is solidity; of apas, contraction; of tejas, expansion; of vayu, motion; and of akasha, pervasion. Prithivi flows midway, apas downward, tejas upward, vayu at acute angles, and akasha transversely. The flow of prithivi tends to endurance; the flow of apas tends to calmness; the flow of tejas tends to death; the flow of vayu tends to motion; the flow of akasha is common to all.

Prithivi is located in the feet, and has a sweet taste. Apas is located in the knees, and has an astringent taste. Tejas is located between the shoulders, and has a pungent taste. Vayu is located in the navel, and has an acidic taste. Akasha is located in the head, and has a bitter taste.

The tattvas are the same in all living things; it is only the arrangement of the nadis that differ. The tattvas function the same in both ida and pingala. In the right nadi, prithivi corresponds to the sun; apas corresponds to Saturn; tejas corresponds to Mars; and vayu corresponds to Rahu, the moon's north node. In the left nadi, prithivi corresponds to Jupiter; apas corresponds to the moon; tejas corresponds to Venus; and vayu corresponds to Mercury.

In the left nadi, ida, the appearance of the breath is that of nectar, as bright as a silvery moon, the great nourisher of the world. The right nadi, pingala, is the motion-imparting force from which the world is continually born. From the sphere of the sun, pingala, poisons such as carbon dioxide exude continuously and go in a stream to the right nostril, just as the lunar fluid of immortality goes to the left. The moon governs sex, the watery parts of the body, the emotions, and the imaginative aspect of both man and woman. The sun governs the creative side, intelligence, and is active and constructive.

The motion of the breath also has a graphic shape, and can tell the aspirant which tattva is active. This may be observed by breathing on water in a shallow vessel or by breathing on a mirror's surface. In the latter case the observation must be made by a second person, for the one who is doing the breathing is too close to the mirror to observe its fleeting impression. In the first example it is the motion of the breath that reveals its form on the water; in the second, the form is produced on the mirror by the vapor of the breath. Prithivi creates a four-cornered shape; apas a semi-circular shape; tejas reveals a triangular shape; vayu a circular form; and akasha creates a spotted effect.

The tattvas can be identified by their color: yellow is prithivi; white is apas; red is tejas (agni); blue is vayu; "spotted" (or that which foreshadows every color) indicates akasha. An aspirant can close his eyes, suspend the breath, and observe the color that comes before his eyes. This can tell him the plexus in which the nerve currents are running, with the most prominent color indicating which chakra is most active. Rarely is a pure color in evidence in the ordinary course of life, as the color of one tattva is always blended with that of other tattvas.

As the breath differentiates in the five tattvic states and chakras it causes varying impressions to come up in the mind. Ida is connected with the left chain of nerves and is the more important in mental development—therefore it is the more important of the two to control through yogic training.

SUBTLE PATTERNS OF BREATH

The ordinary length of the current of air when it is exhaled is about 6 finger-breadths, which is considered to be the normal extent of the flow of vayu. When singing, it increases to 12 finger-breadths; while eating, to 16; when hungry, 20; in normal walking, 18; in sleep, from 27 to 30; in sexual intercourse, from 27 to 36; and in rapid walking or physical exercise it flows even more. Worry produces a whirling breath, making it difficult to talk, while other emotional states affect the breath variously. Decreasing the natural length of the expired air from nine inches to a shorter distance increases one's life span. When the external flow is excessive it makes the internal flow suffer: when the external flow is increased, life is decreased. As long as breath remains in the body, there is life; therefore whatever contributes to keeping prana in the body promotes longevity. When the external length of the breath is sufficiently reduced the aspirant requires no food, and when it is reduced still further it is said that he can fly in the air.

In dreamless sleep, prana sleeps in the blood vessels, the pericardium, and the hollow of the heart. Whenever prana is agitated or in motion, which means in touch with the nadis, ordinary consciousness arises. The greater consciousness that is light, wisdom, and truth, which is latent yet all-pervading, is awakened by the regulation of the motion of prana.

It is important to remain aware of the breath at all times when one is engaged in special activities. By maintaining such awareness the aspirant can make all of these efforts more effective. In time this awareness will become automatic and be of assistance to him in all things. On rising in the morning one should note which nostril is flowing more actively. One should observe the nasal cycle for thirty days and should attempt to make its flow correspond to the patterns mentioned previously. If this is done the subsequent pattern of breathing will correct itself. In the beginning this will be a difficult and demanding process, but soon the breath will abide by the rhythm set for it. Any unusual appetites or restlessness in the body or mind will be corrected when the correct breathing rhythm is established.

If the right breath begins at sunrise on the first day of the bright fortnight (when ideally the left should be active), then there will be some kind of imbalance connected with heat. If the left begins to flow at a time when the right should be active (as at the beginning of the dark fortnight from the full moon to the new moon), then there will be some imbalance connected with cold. Imbalance in the breath can also lead to disappointments and quarrels, and can interfere with all good actions. If this type of disruption in the rhythm continues for three fortnights, the individual will suffer a serious illness. When either nostril flows continuously for a few days the individual is also sure to experience a serious illness soon.

If one feels that a fever is about to come on he should note the nostril in which the breath is flowing and change its course. He should close this nostril and keep it closed until the fever comes down. If the fever is due to cold, the left will dominate; if it is due to heat, then the breath will flow through the right nostril.

The aspirant who can control ida and pingala can certainly control the mind. When the aspirant has control over the flow of ida and pingala and can change their flow willfully, he can then control situations created by the conditionings of the mind. For him there will be no barriers or regression in his progress. The practical aspirant will attempt to keep ida flowing throughout the day and pingala flowing throughout the night.

When ida flows in its proper order toxins are eliminated from the body, while the proper flow of pingala provides strength. The flow in the right and left nostrils determines the functions of ida and pingala during both day and night. The ancient texts indicate that one should breathe through ida all day and through pingala all night. If one can accomplish this his body and mind will remain fresh, he will require little sleep, and he will be resistant to disease. If practiced for three weeks this will become habitual.

Control of the pranas prolongs life. If the flow of the solar breath is kept in check, solar time is effectively controlled and longevity results. Conversely, it is also written that the excessive flow of the breath in ida decreases the life span, and that the restraint of ida lengthens life as well.

The whole science of breath is complex and subtle. For example, the science posits that a day will be auspicious if ida flows both in the morning and at noon, and if pingala flows in the evening. If the solar nostril, pingala, flows at sunrise and then the lunar breath becomes ascendant, that individual will be especially effective in performing his actions. Likewise, it is said that if ida flows at sunrise on the second day of the bright fortnight (when pingala, the solar breath, should flow), then the internal life force begins to work and the individual becomes intuitive.

PINGALA (SUN)

When pingala flows dominantly one should undertake actions that require strength or are normally hard to perform, such as studying abstruse subjects or carrying out strenuous tasks. Traditionally actions such as hunting, climbing trees, harvesting, riding, exercising, swimming in rivers and lakes, climbing hills, or doing strenuous physical work are best undertaken at this time.

The digestive fire and the digestive processes are also enhanced during the flow of pingala. Thus one should eat solids while pingala flows, not while ida predominates. After eating, one should lie on the left side to activate the flow of the right nostril. It is also stressed that one should perform the eliminatory function of defecation when pingala flows. Sleep is also best when pingala is predominant. The flow of pingla is also considered to be the most appropriate for sexual intercourse or all acts which are temporary. Aggressive or negative acts, such as going to war or engaging in fights with enemies, are also said to be best conducted during the flow of pingala. Traditionally it is said that one should not travel in a southerly or westerly direction when pingala flows.

IDA (MOON)

Ida is described as the nostril which should be active when one undertakes all good and prolonged actions. Activities such as traveling long distances (except north and east), beginning to erect monuments or houses, undertaking new studies, planting seeds, accumulating goods, enjoying pastimes, doing charity, or being treated medically are encouraged at that time. It is said, however, that one must also make sure that the proper tattva is working at such times. All acts where calmness of mind is required are said to be best done during the flow of ida. These include marriage and meetings with superiors. The recitation of mantras and the performance of *siddhis* (special yogic powers) are best accomplished during the left flow.

While generally one is encouraged to eat while pingala is active, the texts also indicate that hot or spicy foods, as well as oily, pungent, salty, or sour foods, should be taken when ida flows. It is also said that the body can eliminate toxins from food when ida flows. Taking in liquids and eliminating fluids through urination are both best done during ida's flow.

SUSHUMNA (THE WEDDING OF DAY AND NIGHT)

When the breath appears to flow sometimes through ida and sometimes through pingala, or when both nostrils appear to flow evenly, then one can tell that sushumna is flowing. When sushumna flows the occasion is unsuitable for external actions—only meditation and contemplation should be done. When the breath is in sushumna, intuitive knowledge is received well.

Determining the activity of the tattvas is also important in determining what actions should be done and when. When ida and pingala are flowing fully and the tattva is not congenial, then there can be no success. Success is only to be had when the tattva is congenial to either ida or pingala.

Sandhi is the period when the breath is changing from one nostril to another, and there is a change in the predominant tattva. Determining the status of the tattvas is useful in considering what kinds of acts may be beneficially performed. This knowledge also helps one to avert illness and maintain sound health. The length of the flow of the breath helps one to know which tattva is active: one can detect the length of the flow by feel alone once the comprehensive knowledge of this science is attained.

Beginners use a feather or powder suspended in the air. The tattva can be determined when *khechari mudra* is applied. By applying *yoni mudra* the color of the predominant tattva appears in the mind. One can meditate on the tattvas to assure their full influence and power, and to arrange their flow as one wishes. One's ability to change the tattva depends on his success in lengthening or shortening the breath at will. For example, if the apas tattva is to be brought into action, then the breath should be allowed to flow only 16 fingerbreadths, no more and no less. Success in maintaining the proper regulation of breath requires constant practice.

PRITHIVI TATTVA

Prithivi is the earth tattva and the force of solidity. It is said to enable one to be steady for a long time. It is associated with the muladhara chakra and its color is yellow. The breath forms the shape of a quadrangle when in prithivi. It is said that the flow of prithivi tends to endurance, and that it flows neither fast nor slow. Using the body as a metaphor to describe the tattvas, prithivi is considered to be the feet. Prithivi is said to have moderate motion and slight heat. The force of prithivi flows to the end of the sternum, 12 finger-breadths down. Prithivi rids the body of desire, makes the body substantial, and brings sound health. It causes prana to gradually increase during the day.

The aspirant should do acts which are expected to last a long time when the breath is in prithivi. Prithivi is associated with success, especially when ida is active. In terms of food, prithivi is related to the digestion of sweets. When pingala is in prithivi, one should eat oats or buttermilk. When ida is in prithivi, one is encouraged to take rice, milk, and fruits. Prithivi is also associated with pleasure, growth, affection, playfulness, and laughter. Success is attained in strenuous activities when pingala is active in prithivi.

APAS TATTVA

Apas is the water tattva, and its force is contraction. It is said to make one calm. It is associated with the svadhishthana chakra and its shape is semi-circular or crescent. The color visualized for apas is white. The flow of apas is downward. Apas is associated with the knees. It is a cooling force. It has a rapid motion, and gives success in all good works. Its results are immediate. Apas is said to relieve hunger and thirst and to ameliorate the effects of poisons. The breath in apas moves down 16 finger-breadths to the navel.

Due to apas, prana is increasingly activated during the night. Apas is considered a most auspicious tattva, which should be kept circulating for a considerable time. Apas is associated with success in all acts, especially when the breath is in ida. Temporary or passing acts should be done with apas. With regard to food, apas is involved with fluids and liquids, and is especially associated with the digestion of astringents. One may also take oils in apas. When the breath is in ida, one should take ghee; when in pingala, buttermilk. Apas controls the dosha of kapha. Apas is also associated with pleasure, growth, affection, and laughter.

TEJAS (AGNI) TATTVA

The fire tattva, tejas, is associated with the manipura chakra. Its force is expansion, and the breath in tejas produces an upward-pointed triangular shape. Its color is red. The flow of tejas is upward. This tattva is associated with warmth. It makes the body light and enables one to walk great distances, and control of this tattva enables one to overcome gravity.

The flow of ida in tejas tends toward destruction, death, and decay. Generally this is not an auspicious tattva; it is associated with loss, death, and the performance of harsh acts. Tejas is also associated with fever, trembling, lack of power in the bodily organs, and the process of leaving's one's body. But when pingala flows in tejas, it sustains life. Tejas allows one to consume great quantities of food or drink, and to endure burning heat. When tejas is in ida one should eat fruits. The breath in tejas whirls, is light, and flows down 4 finger-breadths to the chin.

VAYU TATTYA

Vayu tattva is related to the element air and the force of motion. Its chakra is anahata, its color is blue, and its shape is circular. It is localized in the center between the two breasts.

Vayu brings about the reduction of the breath. Vayu is also considered to be generally inauspicious, causing loss and death. The absence of power in the organs, the presence of fever or trembling, and departure from one's body are also associated with vayu. Vayu is considered to be the appropriate tattva for performing ferocious acts, such as those on the battlefield. It gives only fleeting success.

The breath in vayu is either hot or cold in temperature, and it flows down 8 finger-breadths. It also flows at acute angles. Vayu digests acids and is associated with cereals and root foods. When vayu is in ida one should eat vegetables. Vayu tattva controls the vayu dosha.

AKASHA TATTVA

Ether is the constituent of the akasha tattva. Its aspect is pervasiveness, and its shape is described as space punctured with black holes. Its color is described as "spotted" or the color that foreshadows all colors, a kind of opalescence. It is located in the head and flows transversely. Akasha is common to all the tattvas, foreshadows the qualities of all, and is said to try to mix all the tattvas.

Akasha is considered a useless tattva for all acts except higher spiritual practices, in which case it leads to *samadhi*, the deepest state of meditation. It enables the aspirant to hear distant sounds, to have power over the breath, and to know the past, present, and future. Akasha digests the bitter portion of food. One should take salty foods in akasha. When akasha is predominant, a burning sensation is experienced in the breath.

METHODS OF CHANGING
THE FLOW OF THE BREATH

1. When one is awake and it can be done conveniently, one should control his breath by consciously pushing it out and pulling it in slowly through the nostril he wishes to open for as long as he can comfortably.

2. To make the breath flow through one nostril for long periods, a plug of cotton may be used in the opposite nostril. It is best to first make the breath change by pushing and pulling the breath, and then plug the nostril to be closed off.

3. One may lie on one's side and place the hand from that side under the head, which will make the breath flow actively in the opposite nadi.

4. Pressure in the armpit on the side which one wishes to close off will cause the breath to flow in the opposite nostril. This may be done by placing the armpit over a chair or resting it upon a crutch, or by placing a firm pillow in the armpit and pressing it tightly. In India, beginners sometimes carry a short crutch upon which they can lean while seated, so that they may keep the breath flowing in a specific nostril.

5. While sitting down, cross the right leg over the left with the left hand resting on the floor. Then with the middle finger of the right hand press the main nerve of the right great toe at the ankle of that foot for some time, and the breath will change to the right nostril. Reversing the process will make the breath flow in the left nostril.

6. Sit on the floor with one foot flat on the floor, and with the knee bent so that it can be placed in the armpit. Then lean a little to that side so that the knee is pressed

firmly in the armpit. The breath will be forced to flow actively in the opposite nostril from the side pressed.

7. If, while seated on the floor, one hand is placed on the floor and that shoulder is pressed against the wall, the breath can be made to flow in the nostril of the opposite side.

By continued practice one may change the breath very quickly from one side to the other. The time required to change the breath through the above methods will depend upon the strength of the flow in the active nostril. Ten minutes is sufficient in most instances. The pressure must, of course, be properly applied, and this can be determined after a few trials or experiments.

The science of breath is extremely subtle and complex, and requires the aspirant to have a constantly high degree of awareness of mind and body. Developing control over the breath allows one to perform actions in harmony. At an even more advanced level the control of breath allows for the control of prana and helps the aspirant to attain samadhi, in which all opposing forces, dichotomies, and distinctions are transcended and merged into the highest state.

The application of sushumna is very important; without it deep meditation is not possible, and without deep meditation, samadhi cannot be accomplished. To apply sushumna the accomplished yogis concentrate on the bridge between the two nostrils above the upper lip and allow both nostrils to flow freely. Such advanced aspirants do not use any external pressures on any part of the body to change the flow of the breath.

The aspirant who has learned the correct method of meditation and who has control over the wandering of his mind can easily apply sushumna willfully through concentration on the flow of the breath, and can attain samadhi.

The knowledge of *turiya*—the transcendent state of consciousness beyond waking, dreaming, and deep sleep—is easily accessible by applying sushumna. Sushumna application and the awakening of kundalini are two main aims of yoga science.

Without knowing the method of awakening sushumna the joy of meditation cannot be experienced. Pranayama is important in gaining control over the mind, and the application of sushumna is important for deepening meditation. The knowledge of svarodaya is important for maintaining good health and attaining success in the world. Life is complete when the body, breath, and mind are studied comprehensively and the goal of life is attained.

chapter four

DHYANA: MEDITATION

All life comes under the influence of certain cycles. In practicing *dharana* (concentration) and *dhyana* (meditation) it is best to adjust one's practice to certain times in the rhythm of nature. The best periods for concentration and meditation are dawn, dusk, and midnight. The early morning hours between four and six o'clock are especially favorable for intense concentration. At this time the mind and body have been completely rested and all nature is calm. It is at this time that self-unfoldment is best attained. Preparation for meditation consists of bringing the mind to perfect calmness. Never attempt to practice concentration or meditation when under emotional stress or when the breath is disturbed. Do not meditate during the daytime when the right breath, pingala, is flowing, or at night when the left breath, ida, is flowing. During meditation it is important to apply sushumna. Complete silence of the mind is necessary for meditation; the mind should be one-pointed and inward. One should not be sleepy, restless, or in any sort of mental turmoil.

The mind itself can only work well within certain limits of temperature. The greatest mental efficiency occurs at a temperature between 68 and 72 degrees Fahrenheit. The mind cannot be clear and centered when the stomach is filled with food or when the bloodstream is full of nutrients. Food makes the breath heavy, and the mind in turn becomes inert. For serious students of meditation two meals a day is the best routine in the beginning. The student should take only water, juice, or milk in between. Overdoing one's practice is certain to bring about mental dullness and tiredness, and will prevent true progress. Therefore one should be moderate, both in habits and in the practice of meditation.

To gain mastery the student should sit in an asana firmly and without movement. A comfortable and steady pose eliminates physical disturbances and allows the mind to be clear for concentration. Avoid disturbances due to light, sound, and changes of temperature. Control over body consciousness must come first. The head, neck, and trunk should be aligned. The eyelids should be gently closed, without pressure, and the attention should be focused on the point between the eyebrows. The mind should be kept free from all intruding thoughts. If thoughts do intrude, the mind should be brought back to the center of concentration; the breath will then gradually become calm and quietness of mind will follow. By being still the breathing will become serene and regular, and as the practice increases the mind will become calm and steady. When the mind is made tranquil one can attain higher knowledge. In the meditative tradition it is said that if one begins meditative practice by reflecting upon the breath and goes on through the different stages of meditation he will reach perfection.

Whenever the mind wanders—drawn away by various objects, by the senses, or by memory—one should bring it back gently. Whatever thoughts, ideas, or emotions arise in the mind, they are not to be either driven out or allowed to take over: one should simply let them have their play without any effort to direct them and should observe them with detachment when they arise. Before long one will understand the true character and form of the intruding thoughts.

To begin the practice of meditation one must have something on which to focus the mind—an idea, image, or light. If one concentrates by visualizing a light within, he should observe it and follow the light visually, trying to hold it still. When it moves, he should notice its movements. He can also observe the mind when it becomes distracted and wanders from the object of concentration. It is easy to concentrate the mind on an image, for it is natural to form images in the mind. One may visualize an image of a moon the size of a fingernail, about 5½ feet in front of oneself. Another object of concentration is the flow of the breath: one may observe the inhalation and exhalation, focusing on the center between the two nostrils. One should try to avoid any pauses or jerks in the breath and allow it to become calm, serene, and regular. One should practice with determination, sincerity, and consistency, but should not be at all concerned about results.

THE PROCESS OF MEDITATION

If one could maintain a thought steadily without a distraction for five minutes, meditation would result. However, deep states of meditation can be attained by adepts in only one and a half minutes.

Meditation is a practice of focusing *manas*, the sensory mind, and *chitta*, the mind-stuff, without wavering. It is a state whereby *buddhi*, the intellect, closely examines the thought upon which it is concentrated, and develops the ability to discriminate. This state can be attained only through a disciplined mental training, consisting of consciously identifying with the object of meditation. One must be aware of the object of meditation and the unit of thought which is operative at the time, as well as the various stages of consciousness through which the meditator passes. To combine these different features requires a singleness of mind.

In meditation there are three factors: the meditator, the process of meditation, and the object or focus of the meditation. First the awareness of the process is gradually eliminated: with each repetition the object of meditation, which is usually a mantra, becomes increasingly automatic; consciousness of the process decreases until finally one ceases to be conscious of it at all. An ever-increasing ease develops, until at last the repetition is performed quite automatically and quite unconsciously.

Following this the meditator is no longer conscious of himself, because the mind engages and identifies with the object of meditation and dwells in its sphere. Next the mind becomes completely permeated by its constant association with the object. Finally there is the entire disappearance of the object itself and the loss of awareness of one's separateness: the knower, the known, and the knowledge become one. Then there is no play of the mind; nor is there a state of inertia or forgetfulness, but rather a state of absolute consciousness that baffles all attempts at description. When the mind is in a deep meditative state, objective consciousness ceases, and thus investigation and abstract reasoning cannot take place.

Through meditation the aspirant gains confidence, inspiration, and clarity of mind. Pride, lust, ill will, doubt, discontentment, and fear are driven out. One becomes cleansed of dullness, sloth, and all faults, and understands the transitory nature of all things. Finally, meditation puts an end to the cycle of rebirth, and obtains for one all the benefits of renunciation and non-attachment.

Concentration is of three sorts: gross, subtle, and luminous. Gross concentration is that focused upon material objects, an image, or any sort of form. Subtle concentration may be on the flow of the breath. Luminous concentration is that focused on a point of light or an image that is evolved inside the individual.

Through systematic meditation the nature of the mind changes, moving gradually into a higher state of consciousness. Every moment of concentration is a step toward the total absorption of the mind. Gradually one eliminates his attraction to money, fame, power, pride, and false vanity, and becomes absorbed in the glorious great infinity.

Meditation has four phases. In the first there is still an awareness of the differentiation of concrete things. In the second there is an enjoyment and comprehension of universal oneness. In the third stage there is a realization of individual self. The first three stages are "with seed"—that is, there is some subject or object in one's awareness. The fourth state, meditation without seed, is the complete cessation of all movement, in which the essence alone exists. As the process of concentration helps one rise above body consciousness, the process of meditation allows one to rise above the mind.

CONCENTRATION AND
MEDITATION TECHNIQUES

The following practices are used to increase and intensify concentration and meditation. One should remember that no practice should be undertaken without the direct supervision and guidance of an accomplished teacher.

These practices are described only to provide an overview of the diversity and nature of the practices recommended by the scriptures, and many require special preparation and preliminary practices.

A Visualization and Meditation on the Divine in the Heart Center

This exercise is a basic form of meditation. The aspirant should assume his meditative posture, close his eyes gently, and allow the breath to flow smoothly and easily. He next draws upon his imagination to create an attractive image that symbolizes his highest spiritual ideal or concept. For example, one may visualize the image of the Virgin Mary, Christ, the Buddha, Krishna, Moses, or the face of his *gurudeva*. He places this image in his heart, where he surrounds the image with an ocean of light, and holds it there, mentally visualizing it. Any beautiful image may be visualized according to the imaginative capacity of the practitioner.

Some of the original visualizations described in the scriptures are so elaborate that it would require many pages to describe a single image. One must build his mental image as perfectly and completely as possible, and meditate on this alone. He must remain constant in selecting one image and not change from one image to another. Neither should he change his meditative posture from one day to the next.

At first the mind can be held still only for a few moments; it will constantly pursue other ideas. When this happens, one brings the mind back to its focus again and again and continues with the meditation. Eventually one will find the mind becoming less restless. When the mind becomes calm and one-pointed it abstains from brooding on external objects. It becomes inward, subtle, and acquires the ability to penetrate those unfathomable levels that were not known before. A one-pointed mind, when it starts flowing inward, gradually penetrates all the levels of consciousness. For strengthening this ability of the mind the following exercises can be practiced.

Trataka: External Gazing

Trataka is an external concentration practice in which one gazes steadily at some small object without blinking, while the eyelids are held slightly more open than usual. The practice is continued until the eyes strain and water. The eyes should then be closed and rolled gently a few times, then rinsed carefully and gently with cold water. Another method of relaxation involves contracting the muscles around the eyes and then relaxing them. The purpose of this practice is to coordinate the impulses of the sensory and motor nerves, which assists in producing a state of calmness and tranquility necessary for concentration. Trataka preserves and maintains good eyesight, and provides immunity from diseases of the eyes.

During this exercise one makes an effort to consciously cut off each thought at the very moment of its appearance in the mind. One should keep a steady watch for each new thought as it is forming, and stop it there. This will be quite difficult for the mind in the beginning. If the mind cannot be controlled, it should be allowed to flow. One relaxes completely and observes the mind's fantasies, its digressions, and its roaming here and there. As one's practice improves, the stream of ideas, rather than being cut short, will seem to arise even more rapidly. This is an indication that the practitioner is making significant progress and that his mind is becoming clearer and his observation sharper.

This is the actual state of the mind's normal operation, but previously it had not been observed. A state of tranquility is reached when the thoughts seem to arise so fast that they are without number—the attempt to hinder thinking seems to have created more thoughts and more thinking. From this point on one should only act as an observer, letting the mind follow its own course. In this manner it will slow down on its own, and each mental process or operation can be inspected carefully and minutely. The ultimate result will be that the entire movement of the mind is brought under control. The mind may actually suspend itself for a moment. This moment of positive suspension in the mental processes is sufficient to make the aspirant realize his real self.

Various sounds may be heard due to the motion of prana in the nadis. One should not be anxious about these noises, and they may be used for the fixation and concentration of the mind. As the mind becomes absorbed in meditation, these sounds will pass away.

Visions of any sort are merely the product of one's own thought processes and have no independent existence whatsoever. They may also be used as a focus for concentration. One should know that all phenomena that rise in or before his mind are only the products of his own mental world. The student should not allow himself to become involved but should simply observe the process.

Candle Gazing

To perform this practice assume any meditative posture with the head, neck, and trunk comfortably erect. Allow the mind to become calm and collected, and let the breath become serene, even, and regular. Gently open the eyes and gaze fixedly at the flame of a candle placed at a distance of two feet in front of the eyes. Continue to focus on the candle until the eyes water. When this occurs, do not rub the eyes, as this water is impure. Instead close the eyes, make a cuplike shape with the palms of your hands, and place them over the eyes. Then you will see an afterimage of the candle flame. Retain this image, keeping it in your mental vision as long as possible. If it moves up, down, or sideways, try to hold it stationary. It is helpful to move it about willfully. As a result of this practice the eyes are strengthened, making them bright and attractive. The exercise also acts upon the solar plexus and is said to add to one's charm. It is held in high regard as a practice in concentration.

As one continues this practice he will eventually be able to establish this image of the candlelight in the mind's eye without the assistance of the candle. The aspirant will find that he becomes delighted with this image and that he wants to follow after it when it begins to diminish or disappear. When this visualization comes under one's conscious control he may focus on the center of the light and anything he wants to know will be revealed to him as long as his intentions are unselfish.

Various exercises of concentration on light are suggested in the yoga manuals. Concentrating on light between the eyebrows is called subtle concentration. One may also concentrate on an ocean of light in his heart, or on the image of a flame in the region of the navel. Other forms of light may appear from within as a result of the predominance of one tattva or another. The lights of the tattvas are dull, while mental lights are bright. The light of *ojas* (the finest of the primary constituents of the body) is seen when there is no consciousness through the senses. If concentration is done consistently on these lights whenever they appear, one will develop a powerful intentional force or resolve, and a time will come when one will be able to recall these lights at will.

Cultivating the Shadow Man
(Chhaya Purusha Sadhana)

To do this exercise stand in the sun when the sky is perfectly clear so that your shadow appears clearly and distinctly in front of you, approximately 5 to 10 feet in length.

Focus your attention on your shadow at a point at the base of its neck. Hold this view with the eyes steady, the lids slightly opened, for as long as you can. When the eyes become tired and begin to tear, close and open them a time or two, and then raise the head to look into the clear sky. There you will see a figure, a full shadow, which is capable of appearing in many colors. Hold this figure in your concentration for as long as you possibly can. By practicing this exercise regularly the shadow will become transparent, and then you will see two shadows. The first, an outer shell, will appear gradually more transparent, and eventually you will see features on the shadow. Finally these features will turn to face you and you will realize you are looking at yourself. This is a concentration exercise which may be done as a part of your usual practice. This practice may also be done on a moonlit night. It is only suited to those localities where cloudless skies are available for several months of the year.

For an accomplished one, this shadow may be invoked to determine whether it is an auspicious time for certain important events or actions. The shadow man will reveal the state of the tattvas in one's body, which will in turn reveal the secrets of life. The scriptures say that if the practice is done faithfully for twelve years the shadow will be with one both day and night. It will guide him concerning his future and give him insights into the depths of the waking, dreaming, and sleeping states.

After a long time the shadow may be made to appear to the practitioner whenever he wishes. It will rise and leave the body through the portals of the eyes. Then the shadow can be projected upon a screen or wall. When the aspirant can perceive every part of his form in the reflected shadow he obtains perfect control over the breath and beneficial results from all of his acts. Thus seeing his mental body he will develop an understanding of all things about himself. Reaching this stage his passions will become controlled and he will attain enlightenment.

Other Methods of Luminous Concentration (Sukshma Dhyana)

The practice of visualizing one's image by the shadow method is one method of luminous concentration. The method of luminous concentration may also be practiced by fixing one's gaze in space without blinking. When these practices are perfected the yogi attains the capacity to create any sort of picture upon a dark screen in order to see what he desires to know. He also attains the power to visualize kundalini, which cannot otherwise be seen due to its subtlety and great changeability. This, however, takes place only after kundalini is awakened.

In kundalini, the *jiva*, the individual soul, appears in the form of a candle flame, and this may also be used for luminous concentration. In the navel chakra (manipura) resides the solar light related to the fire tattva. Concentrating on this light is called the fire meditation. If the student repeatedly visualizes this light until he becomes aware of it throughout the day and feels as if he is walking in this light, he will be able to realize certain siddhis, or powers of special value.

Another practice involves exhaling completely and then drawing in the solar plexus by uddiyana. One should then practice meditation on the heart center. This practice will awaken the light therein and transmute sexual energy.

Contemplation Upon the Void (Unmani Mudra)

By keeping the attention fixed on a certain idea or by making the mind blank for a sufficient duration, an outgoing of both ideas and will results. The will can thereby inadvertently bring about its own extinction when it is intent upon the extinction of something else, such as an idea.

By the repetition of such a mental action the consciousness of that action grows less, until at last it is performed quite automatically and unconsciously.

One practices this technique to make himself a void so that an influx of the divinity can fill this void with its fullness, as an empty jar is filled by the ocean. One can also direct the pranic energy anywhere one wants in the body by thinking of oneself as hollow inside and sending the thoughts to the place where he wants the current to flow. One should banish all thoughts and be neither inside nor outside the mind. Thus the mind will lose its identity, as salt disappears in water or oil in a fire. The aspirant who practices will be well rewarded, even before this stage is fully achieved, by the attainment of siddhis, such as clairvoyance and the ability to perceive and read the thoughts of others. He who contemplates the void or space while walking, standing, and dreaming will become absorbed in space. An aspirant who desires success should acquire the power of regular and habitual practice, which will produce wonderful results. Such an aspirant will have an experience unlike anything he has ever known before. This feeling is simply indescribable: he will feel like an entirely transformed person, purged of faults and limitations, and living a new life. Such an aspirant becomes beloved by all, and acquires spiritual powers. This is one of the processes of emancipation. By making the mind free and open he himself becomes full, saturated with *sattva*. Even one's normal daily consciousness will be more strongly permeated with awareness than before as a result of the intensity of this practice.

Shambhava Mudra

In this yogic *kriya*, while remaining attentive inwardly to the energy of life in the heart, and with the mind and breath stilled and absorbed, light is directed steadily forward without moving the eyelids. The eyelids are opened as if seeing everything, while actually seeing nothing out-side oneself. This *mudra* brings about the absorption of the mind and a feeling of happiness and joy. To accomplish this mudra, gaze steadily forward into space without seeing anything. Taking your meditative posture, simply gaze fixedly before yourself without attempting to see anything and without blinking the eyelids. The eyelids must be slightly ajar. Adopt a steady stare and contemplate space by rendering the mind void of all thoughts, achieving a state of emptiness. Let no external objects make an impression upon the retina, even though the eyes are wide open.

This practice will bring the breath under control, correct nervous conditions, enable one to overcome fluctuating moods, remedy all undesirable mental states, eliminate self-consciousness, and help one to fully understand what is happening around oneself. When the mind is given this monotonous task, it empties and becomes like a vacuum or magnet: thus the internal world rushes into it. This practice puts the mind in a state of watchful waiting, and truth becomes its natural companion. Those whose sleep has decreased through practice and whose minds have become calm will benefit by performing *shambhava mudra*.

Nasagra Drishti (Nasal Gazing)

In performing this concentration, fix the gaze on the light visualized at the bridge between the two nostrils with the eyebrows raised slightly. Let the mind concentrate on the energy of life in the heart, as in shambhava mudra. One must think of this life energy inwardly, while apparently looking outwardly. This is a good exercise for the wandering mind, if taken up with zest and practiced faithfully for a few months. One should be aware of the flow of the breath in and out of the nostrils. This practice affects the brain through the optic nerve. Initially this should be practiced for brief periods of time, and one should gradually increase the length of the practice period. Those with weak nerves should not undertake this practice without the personal supervision of an expert. This practice is done in siddhasana.

Frontal Gazing

This is an important practice. It is a good exercise for the unsteady mind and a useful preparation for *unmani*. One begins by fixing the eyes on the space between the two eyebrows and allows the eyelids to find their own natural resting place. They will tend to remain slightly open with the whites of the eyes visible. This frontal gaze may be practiced either in siddhasana or in any other meditative posture. As in the nasal gaze, those whose nerves are easily excited must practice with caution.

As a result of this gaze one will be able to visualize the lustre and light from within and his attraction to worldly objects will be eliminated. One must suppress the strong desire that will arise during this practice to open the eyes and to look about for just a moment: this is the action of the physical body seeking to express itself and release itself from the control imposed.

Laya Yoga

This is the absorption of the mind in sound. The goal of this practice is to alter one's normal awareness of self by focusing on hearing an internal, mystic sound. The mind will become steady and absorbed in the sound on which it focuses. In space, sound is produced by the movement of sound waves in the air; so too in the body there are currents that flow and produce sound when one practices pranayama.

To do this practice sit in siddhasana and focus the attention on the spot between the eyebrows. Turn the eyes upward and let the lids remain closed. The eyes, ears, nose, and mouth should be closed. With a calm and controlled mind listen for a sound in the right ear, and eventually you will hear a clear sound. In the beginning the sounds will be very loud and varied, but with continued practice they will become increasingly subtle. At first one may hear sounds that seem to pound and surge, like the beating of a kettle-drum. After some time, in the intermediate stage, the sounds will resemble those produced by a conch shell, or by bells. Finally, after further practice, the sounds will re-semble tinkling noises, the sound of a flute, or the hum of bees. All of these sounds are produced within and cannot be heard by anyone else. One should practice being aware of both the loud and subtle sounds, alternating and vary-ing one's awareness from one to the other, so that the mind will not be inclined to wander.

When the student's mind is intently engaged in listening to these sounds he becomes captivated by them and over-comes all distractions. As a result of this practice the mind gives up its outwardly directed activity and becomes calm, desiring no objects of sense gratification. The mind and breath become refined and one's attention is focused within. Then the yogi forgets all external objects and loses consciousness of himself, and the mind is absorbed in eter-nal bliss. The absorption that is produced when the mind enters the sound *(nada)* emanates spiritual powers and a sort of ecstasy, and one forgets his whole material existence. This absorption is called *moksha*. If one desires to attain the state of union one should practice listening to the *anahata nada*, the unstruck sound, in the heart with a calm and con-centrated mind. When the mind focuses on the sound the mind becomes steady; mental activity is suspended when the mind is absorbed in the sound. The accomplished aspi-rant interpenetrates the anahata sound and attains the state of samadhi through this method of laya yoga.

These internal sounds can be heard only by those whose nadis are free from impurities and who are well practiced in pranayama. The anahata sound comes from sushumna, and, as with other sounds, it cannot be heard by the aspirant until this nadi is free from all impurities. Thus the practice of concentration and absorption with nada (sound) is only possible after considerable preparation. A beginner can instead perform *bhramari*, in which a humming sound resembling a bee drone is produced in one's throat. This practice requires breath control, so that the breath may be exhaled very slowly, producing the sound for a significant length of time.

Just as focusing the awareness on the eyes produces special powers of vision, directing one's awareness to the ears allows one to detect special sounds. By directing the full force of one's attention to these senses the deeper powers develop. Directing the thoughts to any particular sense of the body awakens one's conscious awareness of the powers that correspond to that sense. Concentration upon the organs of the body that are involved in any practice increases their power and sensitivity.

Concentration shows itself in five progressive mental stages: analysis, reflection, bliss, ecstasy, and meditation. The first stage is one of gaining knowledge about the nature of the object. The second step is that of pure reflection; here the lower stage of analysis is transcended. In the third stage the power of reflection gives way to a blissful state of consciousness, which later merges into the pure ecstasy of the fourth stage. In the fifth stage one loses awareness of all sensation, and external awareness gives way to a state of complete meditation. In samadhi there is neither seeing nor hearing, neither physical nor mental consciousness; pure existence is experienced.

chapter five

THE AWAKENING
OF KUNDALINI

Among all the approaches to studying the internal realm, the science of kundalini yoga is the most advanced. The term *kundalini* comes from the Sanskrit word *kundala,* which means "coiled." It is also related to the word *kunda,* a bowl used for sacrificial fires. Kundalini is the primal fire that resides, coiled like a serpent, at the root of the spinal column. This primal energy rests at the perineum in the human body and is symbolized by a shining serpent, coiled three and a half times, with its tail in its mouth, lying as if asleep or dormant. The goal of yoga is to awaken kundalini and to channel this latent energy upward, enabling the aspirant to attain the highest state of consciousness and enlightenment.

The ultimate success of all yoga practices rests upon the awakening of kundalini. The aspirant earnestly seeks to awaken kundalini, which remains asleep in the ordinary person. The mind cannot become one-pointed and concentrated and meditation cannot be successfully practiced until the aspirant awakens kundalini. As long as kundalini remains asleep the individual remains primitive and true knowledge does not arise. But with the awakening of kundalini the deadening covers and shackles of matter are removed. He who moves this shakti enters the path that releases one from all bondage. Awakening kundalini is a highly systematic method of attaining self-realization, in which intense practice over a long period of time is necessary.

Sincerity, truthfulness, solitude, and self-discipline are necessary prerequisites on this path. Exercises to awaken the kundalini energy should be practiced only under the guidance of a teacher who is a master of this science. Those who have not purified their minds and become selfless may bring harm to themselves and others if they attempt to misuse this high spiritual energy for their own material or ego-centered goals. Those who are not prepared physically, emotionally, and mentally for this increased energy may come to harm if they attempt to practice this science only through reading books.

To truly understand kundalini yoga one must study the subtle philosophy of tantra. The foundation and core principle of tantric philosophy is the understanding that the entire universe is a manifestation of pure consciousness, and that nothing exists separate from this consciousness. The goal of the system of tantra is to lead the aspirant toward the realization of this pure consciousness, both within and without. According to the philosophy of tantra the world is not created from matter separate from this highest consciousness. Rather, the world is a manifestation or expression of consciousness, and consciousness is inherent in all manifestations.

In the process of manifestation, consciousness divides itself into two aspects, neither of which can exist without the other. One aspect retains a static quality and remains identified with unmanifested consciousness. In tantra yoga this quality is called *shiva* and is conceptualized as masculine. Shiva is depicted as being absorbed in the deepest state of meditation—a state of formless being, consciousness, and bliss. He remains aloof to the manifestation of the universe. Shiva has total power to be, but no power to become; alone, he has no power of manifestation. Yet consciousness, as the power that manifests the whole world, arises out of this source.

The other part of this polarity is a dynamic, energetic, and creative aspect that is called *shakti*. Shakti is the great Mother of the Universe, and it is from her that the forms, objects, and material creation are manifested. Shakti is the subtlest energy and power of the universe. She manifests herself as all matter, energy, the mind, and the life force in all creatures. Shakti is a projection of consciousness that veils the pure consciousness from which she was projected. Her innumerable illusory manifestations, termed *maya,* bring forth that which is called the universe. When the universe is dissolved it is drawn back into shakti, to the same source that is the basis of its creation. The two principles of shiva and shakti are eternally and inseparably united, but an illusion of separation is created between pure consciousness and its power of manifestation.

Energy exists in two forms: dynamic and latent. All activities or forces of motion have a static background, and when consciousness manifests itself as the creative or dynamic principle it divides itself into these two aspects. The dormant force that supports the whole universe is symbolized by the serpent-like, coiled-up energy.

In tantric philosophy a human being is seen as being like a miniature universe or a microcosm that parallels the whole of the external manifestation, the macrocosmic universe. The principles that govern the universe also govern every individual. Thus the human microcosm contains all of the constituents of the external world: earth, water, fire, air, and ether. The system of tantra emphasizes the subtle connections between the external universe and the human microcosm. It often uses a poetic and subtle symbolism, in which these two universes are compared, when it describes various practices for awakening kundalini. In this way the more advanced techniques are shielded and protected from unprepared aspirants, who do not understand this subtle symbolism.

Kundalini is the highest manifestation of consciousness in the body. It represents the creative force of the world as manifested in human beings. Kundalini is creative energy in a static state, the spiritual force itself, "the Grand Potential," the residual power. Kundalini embodies all powers and all forms. Therefore she is the seat of all physical and mental manifestation. There must be a static background in any sphere of activity or of energy: thus the bodily forces necessarily presuppose some static support. The pranic forces are but the motion of kundalini, the static center of the whole body. Kundalini is the center for all manifestations of energy. All the forces that emanate from this source traverse the whole body and then return, just as electricity runs out of the positive pole of a battery and returns to it by way of the negative pole. This is the center of manifestation of all the forces that act in the living human frame.

Kundalini is said to be the mother or origin of the three qualities, or *gunas* (attributes of *prakriti*): *sattva, rajas,* and *tamas. Sattva* means "existence, light, and illumination"; *rajas* means "activity"; and *tamas* refers to "darkness, the obstructing quality." Kundalini is the fountainhead of energy and knowledge. From the seat of kundalini the mind is born, as is the physical vessel, the body. From the seat of kundalini the fire of life is augmented: from this source arise the *vayus* (the energies within the body), *bindu* (the seed of life), and *nada*, or sound, the very source of speech. Kundalini is not an object of visualization, but a most subtle entity in the form of light. She is the power from which all nature's gifts proceed. Just as all the powers of this universe exist in God, so do all the powers of the individual exist in kundalini. It is this shakti that lies at the foundation of the wonders performed by yogis.

Manifest energy has three aspects: neutral, centripetal (toward the center), and centrifugal (away from the center). In the nervous system centripetal currents are called sensory or afferent currents; centrifugal currents are called motor or efferent currents. These currents exist in their neutral state in kundalini at the muladhara chakra. Nutrition and oxygen are taken into the body by the centripetal currents; carbon dioxide and other wastes are expelled by the centrifugal currents. The vital force is the foundation and origin of all manifestations of the physical energy and must not be mistaken for the functions of the brain, heart, or any other part of the body that it creates: by doing so, we would confuse the creative force with that which is created.

In the system of tantra the human body is seen as a reservoir, with vast quantities of energy that are not used for the purposes of maintaining human life. It is this untapped energy that is symbolized as the serpent, kundalini, resting in her abode at the base of the spinal column. This energy is the static support of the entire body and all its pranic energies. It is the divine force in the human body. Prana, the dynamic aspect of energy that provides the working force for the body, evolved from that energy of shakti. As electrical energy is more subtle than mechanical energy, pranic energy is more subtle than electrical energy. This energy, the way it functions, and the channels it uses for its functioning have been studied thoroughly in yogic science.

THE CHAKRAS

The vital force of shakti in the body is organized around specific centers. These are not physical centers, but they do have physical correspondences to the various plexuses of the body. These energy centers, called *chakras,* help organize the physical body, although they cannot be perceived by means of the bodily senses and organs.

It is necessary for the aspirant to have a clear and comprehensive knowledge of the chakras before he begins treading this path of inner light. Yoga science is very complex and extensive. It includes the study of the body, the nervous system, and the life forces that govern bodily functions. In addition it includes careful study of the mind, its modifications, and all states of consciousness, as well as the philosophy of the universe and of human relationships. Tantra philosophy integrates all these levels of knowledge. In order to reach an integral understanding of all these, the student of tantra studies the chakras, their nature, and their interrelationships. He also finds it necessary to know all the sheaths, or bodies.

Within the *annamaya kosha,* the physical body, is the *pranamaya kosha,* the pranic body or energy sheath—and more subtle still is the *manomaya kosha,* the mental body. After carefully examining the human being in his totality one realizes that matter, energy, and mind are not the whole of human existence. Beyond these three lies the self-existent principle of pure consciousness. The external body (the physical sheath), its energy (the pranic sheath), and the mind (the mental sheath) all veil and conceal the light of consciousness. These bodies, or sheaths, do not function independently; they are connected and coordinated by the chakras.

There are seven major chakras that are important for understanding kundalini. The manifestation of the cosmic force is expressed through these centers, which energize and govern corresponding regions of the body. Kundalini is manifested in the form of each center. The result is a particular frame of reference through which the individual experiences the world. For example, when the mind and energy are expressed through *anahata chakra*, the heart chakra, one becomes compassionate and is able to control emotional energy.

The chakras are located along the central axis of the body in conjunction with the spinal cord. Energy is usually focused in one or more of these centers to the relative exclusion of others. Differences in where energy is focused from person to person, and from time to time, help to account for differences in the way the world is experienced from one individual to the next, and from one moment to the next.

The two lowest centers may be grouped together because they represent the most primitive expressions of energy and states of consciousness that are most closely tied to the physical world. They are linked to the basic instincts for the survival of the individual and of the species. When energy is focused in these centers, pure consciousness is obscured and the individual identifies with the grossest material plane of existence. These chakras have the quality of tamas (inertia).

The next two chakras, located at the solar and cardiac plexuses, represent a turning to more subtle relationships with the world. Here one attempts to organize and make sense of the world and to interact on a less physical plane than in the case of the first two chakras. There is a focus on the building up and expansion of one's sense of I-ness. The predominant characteristic is that of rajas (expansion and activity).

The fifth and sixth chakras, which correspond to the cervical and pituitary centers in the human body, represent a movement away from worldly relationships to a world of purity. Here one perceives and relates to the underlying forms from which the material universe comes.

One who is operating at these levels exhibits creativity, intuition, and wisdom. His manner is predominantly sattvic (serene and devotional). There is a series of still more subtle chakras above the pituitary center (the *ajna chakra*), culminating in the center of pure consciousness at the crown of the head. This is the abode of shiva, pure transcendent consciousness. This center is named *sahasrara*.

Ordinarily shiva and shakti are separated, with shiva residing at the crown of the head and shakti (kundalini) resting dormant at the base of the spine. Only the smallest bit of shakti's energy becomes dynamic and functions in the chakras and nadis in order to maintain the functions of the ordinary individual. Those who awaken this force from its latent to its active form become the dynamic geniuses of every age and culture.

The place or seat of kundalini is *muladhara chakra*, at the perineum. The muladhara chakra is about four finger-breadths square, with its face toward the posterior. This space is called the root, and from here arise 72,000 nadis. Here kundalini, self-illumined, is haloed by a golden light. It lies in a lethargic state, coiled three and a half times, and covers the entrance of sushumna (brahma nadi) with its face. The object of yoga is to make this vital force, kundalini, move in sushumna—which she otherwise obstructs, thus hindering the breath from entering there. The ultimate goal is to allow the kundalini force to reach *brahmarandhra*, the thousand-petaled lotus. The fontanel is the end point of kundalini on its way through sushumna.

The practice of kundalini yoga involves not only awakening kundalini shakti but also systematically leading her through each of the chakras to the crown chakra (sahasrara), the abode of shiva. The word *yoga* means "union," and this union can be understood as the uniting of kundalini shakti with shiva (pure consciousness). When the individual attains this state he becomes fully conscious. There is no longer an unconscious or latent power—the individual is fully awakened and illumined. When the static shakti becomes dynamic and travels upward, fully energizing each of the centers along the way, the polarization of the body gives way and one attains the highest state of samadhi. Consciousness of the body is withdrawn.

As a static power kundalini sustains consciousness of the world—but when she unites with shiva one loses consciousness of the world and goes to a state of consciousness without object or form. When she is aroused and moves upward, kundalini withdraws into herself the dynamic forces that maintain the body. This is the reverse of involution, of consciousness involving itself in the universe: it is a process of evolution, in which the human being comes to realize his full potential. The final goal of the aspirant is to abide in that state of pure consciousness. While in this state, outwardly the body may no longer seem to be alive, but it continues to function minimally, so that it can again be used as an instrument by the individual who has temporarily left it. The union of shiva and shakti generates a nectar that continues to sustain the body in this superconscious state. This union is the supreme goal of the aspirant, but only a fortunate few achieve it. It is more common, although still rare, for the aspirant to awaken kundalini shakti and lead her only part of the way toward her goal.

In order to understand the spiritual evolution and transformation of the aspirant it is important to understand the chakras fully, since the energy focused in the chakras determines the personality and level of awareness of the individual. As the aspirant evolves, his personality becomes gradually more refined and purified.

The first chakra is at the perineum, between the genitals and the anus, the starting point of *chitrini nadi*. This is also the location of the mouth or opening of sushumna. The *kanda,* or root, from which all the subtle nadis originate is found here; sushumna comes out of the kanda. This chakra is *muladhara,* the root support chakra. Muladhara is the earth region and is represented by a square surrounded by four lotus petals at the four corners of the square. These petals symbolize four *vrittis* (modes of consciousness). The *bija* (seed sound vibration) of this chakra is *lam.* The color yellow and the sense of smell are manifestations of muladhara. Psychologically, this center is related to the instinct for individual survival. Until one gains mastery over this chakra, insecurity, fear, and paranoia are the major emotions and attitudes associated with it. The terror of total annihilation disturbs one at this level and colors his view of the world. Individuals whose level of awareness is focused at this center see the world as a jungle where they need to fight for their very existence. Those who are integrated at this center have feelings of stability, security, and groundedness.

The second chakra, *svadhishthana,* is situated within the section of the vertebral column corresponding to the genital area. More specifically, svadhishthana is found at the upper border of the triangular piece of bone in the spinal column that is wedged in between the two hip bones known as the sacrum. This abode is about halfway between the navel and sex organ and some nine inches above the seam of the perineum. *Svadhishthana* means "her own abode." This is the center of kundalini's original abode, before she became intoxicated and fell to the muladhara chakra, where she is said to lie in a coiled, dormant state. Svadhishthana chakra has six petals, whose color is vermillion. These represent the six vrittis of indulgence, the absence of empathy, destructiveness, delusion, disdain, and suspicion. At the center, which is creamy white in color, is a water region in the shape of a crescent moon where the bija *vam* is found. Svadhishthana is responsible for the sense of taste. This center is concerned with issues of sensuality and sexuality. Individuals whose energy is expressed from this chakra view the world from the perspective of pleasure gratification, particularly sexual pleasure, and feelings of lust or repression prevail. Here one is absorbed in the polarity of masculinity and femininity; integration yields a sense of androgyny and an appropriate, controlled expression of sexuality. The tantric texts say that one who achieves mastery over this chakra is free from all enemies and becomes like the sun, removing the darkness of ignorance with his light. His words flow like nectar in expressing the wealth of his wisdom.

The third chakra is found in that part of the vertebral column corresponding to the solar plexus. It is called *manipura*, meaning "filled with jewels." There are ten lotus petals at manipura, indicating the following vrittis: spiritual ignorance, treachery, jealousy, shame, delusion, disgust, fear, foolishness, discontent, and sadness. At the center of manipura is a triangle the color of fire. At the center of this fire region is the root sound of fire, *ram*. The sense of sight arises from this chakra. This center determines the assimilation of food, and digestive disorders may indicate unresolved issues at this level. Psychologically, this is the center of the ego. It brings out one's concerns with power and competition: issues of domination and submission and of aggression and passivity arise from this chakra. Integration at this level leads to assertiveness, cooperation, and dynamic energy.

The *anahata chakra* is located between the breasts in the region of the heart. *Anahata* means "unstruck sound." Intense concentration at this chakra may lead one to hear the sound of bells within. The anahata chakra divides the body into two hemispheres: the upper and the lower. The three centers below the diaphragm represent the primitive expression of consciousness, and are concerned with the gross instinctual aspects of human beings. They are closely related to the physical and sensual world and the desire to obtain pleasure-giving objects. Negative emotions arise out of those centers, and dwelling at those levels indicates a lower level of human nature. But when consciousness rises above the horizon of the diaphragm one becomes truly human and higher consciousness dawns. It is at this center that the upward- and downward-moving forces meet. That is why it is considered to be a center of equilibrium. The anahata chakra motivates one to be active and rajasic, but at the same time it is considered to be a center that gives emotional maturity and leads one toward sattva.

Anahata is symbolized by a twelve-petaled lotus representing thought forms to be dealt with at the center. Within the lotus are two interlaced triangles, one pointed upward and the other downward, and at the center is the bija *yam*. This center is related to the element air and the sense of touch. Its color is smoky grey. Anahata is the center from which one feels unconditional love toward others, and seeks to offer nurturance and service. Compassion, selfless love, and empathy are the attributes of this chakra. Just as the heart and lungs nourish the entire body and the mother's breasts nurture the baby, one who has attained this level nurtures others. Here one passes beyond the sense of isolation from others that characterizes the experience of the lower chakras.

The fifth chakra is located in the vertebral column at the hollow of the throat. It is called the *vishuddha chakra*, which means "purified." Here there are sixteen lotus petals. Each contains one of the sixteen vowel sounds of the Sanskrit alphabet and represents a quality that is cultivated with mastery over this chakra. The *akasha* principle—space, ether, or the void—is the force of this chakra. The color of vishuddha is blue and its bija is *ham*. The sense of hearing is controlled by this center. Vishuddha is the seat of receptivity and creativity. Devotion, surrender, trust, and willingness are qualities that it engenders. Musicians and artists are said to have their energy concentrated here.

The sixth chakra is located at the space between the eyebrows at the "third eye." The chakra is not actually on the surface of the forehead but is within the sushumna where it passes through the brain at the level of the space between the eyebrows. This center is called the *ajna chakra,* which means "command." The ajna chakra has two lotus petals, one on each side, in which the *matrika* letters *ha* and *ksha* are found. This center is also called *tripatha sthana,* the terminal of the three lines of power: ida, pingala, and sushumna. The qualities of introspection and discriminative intellect are related to this center. One who has mastered this level has inner vision, sees all things clearly, and acquires higher intuitive knowledge and wisdom. He has attained sushumna by integrating the right and left polarities, pingala and ida, and thus develops both logical judgment and intuition to their fullest. The mantra of this chakra is *Om:* when one has attained mastery of this center the mother of all mantras is heard within.

Meditation on vishuddha and ajna, which correspond to the cervical and pituitary centers, awakens spirituality and leads one to obtain the experiences of the inner world. Creative intelligence, wisdom, and intuition arise from these two chakras, which have the quality of the sattva guna. There are many subtle chakras above the ajna chakra, culminating in the seventh major chakra, the center of pure consciousness, at brahmarandhra, the soft spot at the crown of the head. This chakra is called the thousand-petaled lotus, *sahasrara*. This is the abode of shiva, of pure consciousness. One who has attained this level is in a state of samadhi. Here the individual self and the cosmic self merge.

While shiva and shakti are separated, kundalini shakti lies dormant at the base of the spine, and only a small part of the energy of kundalini is available for one's use. The rest of this energy remains in a potential form. Human beings remain ignorant because they are not aware of this vast reservoir of energy, and they are not able to use it for the attainment of the purpose of life. Those who are capable of transforming kundalini from its latent to its active stage become dynamic. If one is dynamic in any avenue of life it is because of the power of shakti or kundalini.

The transforming experience is possible only after awakening kundalini in a systematic manner, under the guidance of a teacher who knows the subject both practically and theoretically. Usually this transformation is depicted as a sudden, intense, and "earthshaking" experience. But such an experience is rare. It is more usual for bits of this energy to be released through various means. One then experiences breakthroughs, bursts of energy and enthusiasm, peak experiences, a sense of well-being, and similar changes in consciousness. Occasionally there are more startling breakthroughs, in which a significant quantity of the latent power is released.

One must not only awaken but also systematically lead kundalini through each of the chakras to the abode of shiva, the sahasrara chakra. According to tantric literature, this union is the highest. When the aspirant is able to achieve this union he becomes fully aware of all the dimensions of life, and he is illumined. One goes through a process of evolution in which he comes to realize his own essential nature and he then abides in that state of pure consciousness.

PREPARATION FOR
AWAKENING KUNDALINI

With the help of a competent teacher the aspirant can awaken the sleeping kundalini and lead it to the final abode of shiva, thus attaining the union of the individual self and the Self of all. It is important to emphasize that a competent teacher will not encourage the student to develop special abilities or powers, such as clairvoyance, because they are only side paths: pursuing these as goals leads one off the main path of enlightenment. A teacher who brags about or attempts to profit from such special abilities can only hamper the student's progress and should be avoided.

When teachers work with students today they often discover that students create many barriers to their growth with habits, attitudes, and practices. The tantric tradition is highly systematized and organized. It is imperative that the student systematically follow the basic instructions and master the preliminary practices before the teacher can lead him to more advanced practices, or the student can be harmed mentally, physically, or emotionally. Thus realized teachers stress that the student must master certain essential steps, and then they watch and wait for the student to prepare himself for more advanced lessons.

First the student must work with his physical body to achieve and maintain a level of health that allows him to concentrate seriously and faithfully on his practices. One must overcome laziness and develop the ability to regulate his habits so that the body does not become a barrier to his progress. He should avoid extremes in food, sleep, and sexual activities to keep the body balanced and healthy. Some misguided students have the unfortunate idea that drugs can lead one on the path of enlightenment, but the use of such substances will disorganize them and hamper their growth.

Next the student must work to refine his personality so that selfishness, pettiness, and egotism do not hold him back on the path. He must cultivate patience, faithfulness, and determination. Many students today begin their practices and soon become impatient: they either abandon their practices, jump from one practice to another, or entirely change their path. Such unsteadiness will not allow one to progress. The modern student thinks that if he is not having dramatic or extraordinary experiences his mantra must be wrong or that there could be a better teacher or practice. He seeks a new mantra or a new teacher. But if one repeatedly switches his practice he will make no progress. Another kind of student does not practice regularly—yet he expects extraordinary experiences to dawn without any effort.

The majority of students today expect to have their kundalini awakened by teachers and gurus rather than through their own efforts. Students sometimes claim that their kundalini was raised by a teacher's gaze, touch, or presence. Such students mistake the body's shakiness, jerks, or other movements, which indicate physical or emotional imbalance, for the movement of kundalini. Emotional reactions and hallucinations are also mistaken for valid experiences. Teachers who encourage such superficial experiences mislead their students. To genuinely awaken kundalini one must first prepare himself, and then patiently and with faithfulness and determination carry out his practices. In this way he will definitely progress. A number of specific methods have been developed to help the student awaken the sleeping kundalini force. The competent teacher selects the method appropriate for each student according to the student's capacities, inclinations, and level of attainment.

To genuinely awaken kundalini one must first prepare himself. Without long and patient practice in purifying oneself and strengthening one's capacity to tolerate and assimilate such a flood of energy, the awakening of this latent power would deeply disturb, disorient, and confuse the student. Even at the physical level such a charge of energy can threaten the integrity of the body. Only after one has developed considerable self-control can this charge be tolerated without the organism's being strained to the point of danger. With careful training the aspirant can gradually come to recognize and master his unconscious demons—in other words, he can purify and strengthen himself. Then, and only then, is he prepared to face the full awakening of all that is latent within him. However, if the aspirant has not purified himself through various spiritual practices, the battle that is waged within can be especially intense, even unbearable. Releasing kundalini without preparation is like opening Pandora's box without having cultivated the ability to master what emerges. For this reason a competent teacher makes sure that the student is prepared.

KUNDALINI AWAKENING

As a key unlocks a door, yoga practices awaken kundalini and open the door to Brahman, the Absolute. When kundalini is aroused it is only a matter of time and practice until all the chakras are penetrated in successive stages, thus giving life and action to these subtle centers in the spinal column. Kundalini can pierce these chakras and pass through brahmarandhra, where it becomes free from all gross forms. Sushumna then becomes the main route for the passage of prana. The mind can then be completely controlled. Kundalini leaves the entranceway to sushumna and begins to move into it as soon as the yogi stops breathing. When the breath passes through sushumna, the central nadi, a state of mental absorption is produced.

Kundalini normally derives her sustenance through pingala in the morning and evening, sleeping at all other times. Through special postures and the practice of kumbhaka and mudras, kundalini is awakened, sushumna becomes free of its impurities, and the mind becomes absorbed in samadhi. When kundalini is fully awakened the aspirant can enter samadhi any time he wishes. He gains supremacy over his body and can withdraw his awareness from sensation, bringing the passions and emotions under complete control. Seminal production and reabsorption can be perfectly balanced only after the full awakening of kundalini. Eventually one acquires the power of arresting all vital bodily functions. In the more advanced stages the entire body sinks into a state of dormancy which resembles that preceding death.

The heat generated by kumbhaka, when coupled with special controls, moves this storehouse of energy into action. Jalandhara bandha and mula bandha check the downward tendency of apana. Ashvini mudra makes apana go upward. Uddiyana bandha makes the united force of prana-apana enter sushumna. Through *shakti chalana* one forces the kundalini from muladhara upward through the plexuses—that is, by uniting prana and apana (pulling apana to the place of prana, and simultaneously forcing prana to the place of apana, moving at one time through ida and at another time through pingala alternately) kundalini is moved from its resting place.

Once one has perfected pranayama he should practice maha mudra, one of the most important means of awakening kundalini shakti. First the physical, organic action is stopped, followed by the development of absorption and complete suspension of animation. Thus all inner and outer forces are subdued and the mind identifies itself with its source, the individual life force. In following this practice one must first observe a strict diet, and must abstain from sexual intercourse for at least a month. A diet of rice, milk, pure cane sugar, barley broth, and fruits will hasten one's accomplishment.

MANTRA

Kundalini is both light and sound, and the techniques of mantra yoga are also used to arouse kundalini. Mantra yoga is one of the branches of tantra and is an effective way to awaken this fountainhead of knowledge. The term *mantra* refers to the practice of uttering special formulas composed of certain sounds or chants with special meanings. There are three ways to remember mantras: with sound expressed through the vocal cords, silently, and mentally. One can gain the greatest power from a mantra by constant mental repetition. Either external or silent repetition of mantra may help the student to some degree, but one never attains the higher powers of mantra by such practice. The mental process of repetition is difficult to understand without the guidance of a competent teacher. Fasting for three to seven days usually precedes the use of mantra to awaken kundalini. Then by constant prolonged repetition of the mantra with feeling and concentration, the mantra consciousness is awakened and the power of the mantra (siddhi) is attained.

Mantra is endowed with the powers of action and sensation, and as such it circulates through the body protecting the vital airs (vayus). Mantra is manifested as a subtle energy and may appear as a flame of fire to the aspirant. Sometimes the flame rises up, and other times it settles down into the apas tattva of the svadhishthana chakra.

The almost imperceptible sound of the flow of the breath is also a mantra. This is the mantra *hamsa. Ham* is the outward flow and *sa* the inward motion. The jiva, the individual soul, has its support in *hamsa*. This mantra is uttered 22,600 times every twenty-four hours.

In this context the term *bija mantra* means seed mantra, and refers to the potential energy that rests in each chakra. As we have seen, a special bija is connected with each chakra. The bija mantra that resides in the muladhara chakra of kundalini is called "self-born." The mantras of the muladhara, manipura, and ajna chakras are used to awaken and attain control in these respective centers. When a mantra has been practiced for a long time it becomes automatic. Each mantra has a form, or *devata*. When the mantra becomes automatic the devata wells up in the heart like a flash of intuition. Eventually the devata will appear visibly before the yogi.

The sensory organs—such as those involved in sight, hearing, and taste—respond to vibrations within certain limits. When the limits are exceeded the organs remain insensitive to these vibrations or impulses. A nervous stimulus brings about a change in the nerve by creating a reaction in it. This change may be slight after the first stimulus, but each repetition of the stimulus increases the reaction, until by constant repetition a permanent alteration may occur in the nervous matter stimulated. The breath brings about such a change in the function of the nervous energy as a result of the practice of mantra.

When a yogi fixes his attention on a mantra and does it faithfully 100,000 times or more he attains siddhi, and all his desires are granted. Even one who is heavily burdened with the results of past actions may attain success by mantra yoga if he repeats the mantra 200,000 times. One gains the power of attracting others who remain always under his influence and protection when his practice is done 300,000 times. One becomes a vehicle for power when the mantra is repeated 600,000 times. Each accomplishment gives added power and perfection.

Siddhis, or higher powers, come to an aspirant when he has his prana and mind under control. When siddhis begin to take form, phenomena may appear before the mind in the various forms of mist, smoke, hot air, wind, fire, fireflies, lightning, crystal, or the moon. Each of these are experiences or stages on the path to siddhis. Siddhis are spoken of as being like possessions: they are not to be sought after, lest they become obstructions to the aspirant.

In the same manner that a man may dote on his wealth, so that the wealth becomes a great preoccupation for him, constricting his consciousness, so also may siddhis become hindrances. They may expose the possessor to his own egoistic and destructive tendencies and may lead to spiritual regression if he uses these siddhis wrongfully. Siddhis are not harmful in themselves, but they may become so when they are abused or become the instruments of wrongful actions. On the other hand they are a wonderful stimulus to progress if kept secret and used only on the most carefully considered occasions.

FURTHER METHODS
TO AWAKEN KUNDALINI

1. Sit in siddhasana with a soft ball or pad of cotton placed so that it exerts pressure on the space between the sex organ and the anus. Then practice khechari mudra, in which the tongue is curled back and placed against the palate. The eyes are focused between the eyebrows, and kumbhaka is done, followed by jalandhara. Then one contracts the anus and navel and presses the breath to the lower end of sushumna in-

stead of letting it go to ida or pingala. The agni will then flame up due to the flowing of vayu, which enables kundalini to pierce the primary nadi, sushumna, after which it can be made to open all chakras. When sushumna is active one feels an ascension of the fire to the brain, as if a hot current of air were being blown through the channel from the bottom to the top. The muladhara and svadhishthana chakras tremble with the force that travels through the body, and kundalini becomes absorbed with shiva. When one attempts to awaken kundalini by this method he should always keep her in his mind and should think of her as extending to the tip of the tongue. He should pay homage to her with every bit of food and drink he takes.

2. Using a bandage, secure a cotton ball against the perineum. Sit with the legs extended forward, and keeping the legs stiff with the feet slightly apart, place the head on the knees, grasping the great toes with the thumbs and forefingers, and bring the trunk down to a position parallel to and as close to the thighs as possible. Inhale through the left nostril and do kumbhaka with tension on the anus and navel, pulling them together, which forces prana into the sushumna nadi. When fatigued, exhale through the right nostril and then do a similar process from right to left, finishing with an exhalation through the left nostril.

3. By applying the navel lock (uddiyana bandha) for 1½ hours kundalini is drawn up a little. This causes it to leave the entrance of sushumna. With the thumb and fingers of each hand, place one hand on each side of the body near the navel and hold the ribs firmly. Now move the stomach with a motion from right to left, and then left to right (nauli), stirring up kundalini. This must be done fearlessly for about 45 minutes.

4. To force kundalini into sushumna she must be stimulated for 1½ hours. This can be done by doing bhastrika and then nauli, which, in time, will cause her to come to life. If this practice is continued for 40 minutes each day one can awaken kundalini within a year. Further time may be required due to impurities in the nadis. One should not despair if it requires a little more time to obtain results. Some physical pain must be endured in this practice. Always begin your practice with a few rounds of bhastrika.

5. The following practice will reduce the time of awakening kundalini. A cloth of soft material of a size that will allow it to be folded a number of times to make a pad about nine inches across and about four inches thick is placed against the navel and tied in this position with some sort of band. During this practice many renunciates cover their bodies with ashes, especially over the heart, stomach, and the region of the sex organs. Then, assuming siddhasana, suspension is done followed by jalandhara, uddiyana, and ashvini. A greater contraction is put on the rectum, and then the abdomen is pushed in and out as in uddiyana, and nauli is practiced until kundalini starts moving.

   If this practice is done for 40 minutes each day kundalini should be brought to life within one year. Perspiration that results from this practice should always be rubbed back into the body. Exhalation must never be done hastily, and one should not carry kumbhaka to such a point that he needs to exhale quickly. The eyes should be focused on the bridge between the nostrils or at a point between the eyes, and one should mentally visualize a flame in the region of kundalini.

6. The practice of shakti chalana mudra is used to awaken kundalini from her sleep in the muladhara chakra. The

fire in this chakra is increased by the flow of apana vayu, and kundalini is energized and begins to move through sushumna. Assume the *baddha padmasana* (bound lotus) posture or sit in siddhasana. Inhale through the right nostril, do jalandhara, and focus the eyes on the bridge of the nose or between the eyebrows. Suspend the breath in the svadhishthana chakra, contract the rectum (ashvini mudra), and draw in the navel (uddiyana). Before the suspension has weakened, exhale very slowly through the left nostril. Repeat this process several times. In this way the serpent-like kundalini, feeling suffocated, awakens and rises upward. This practice is followed by yoni mudra. When one begins to perspire he should rub the perspiration over the body.

7. Another technique used by those accomplished in breathing practices is to draw in the breath with short gasps until the lungs are distended, the left more so than the right. Then one presses the body so as to apply pressure to the heart. This leads to the attainment of perfection in pranayama more effectively than any other method.

OTHER PRACTICES

Anahata Nada

This exercise should be practiced in the middle of the night when there is no sound to be heard. The yogi should practice kumbhaka, closing his ears with the two thumbs, the eyes with the index fingers, the nostrils with the middle fingers, the upper lip with the ring fingers, and the lower lip with the little fingers. Firmly confining the air, he should listen attentively for sounds in his right ear. These sounds will gradually be recognized if one practices daily. The aspirant loses body consciousness and becomes one with the higher self. Through regular practice the aspirant progressively hears ten distinct sounds. The first is like the hum of the honey-intoxicated bee; the second, like a bamboo flute; the third, the ringing of bells; fourth, the sound of a conch shell; fifth, the sound of a stringed instrument; sixth, a silver cymbal; seventh, a kettledrum; eighth, a clay drum or trumpet blast; ninth, thunder. The tenth and last sound that is heard is the anahata sound rising from the heart. This last sound has a resonance, in which there is a light. The mind should be focused on this light. When the mind becomes absorbed in this light one attains a higher state of wisdom. For those who do not tread the path of knowledge the practice of *anahata nada* is recommended. Among the many methods for obtaining the state of absorption, the practice of anahata nada is said to be the best.

Bhramari (Bee-Droning) Kumbhaka

While seated in a tranquil posture, the yogi begins to breathe through both nostrils slowly, gradually increasing his respirations and making them more and more frequent, until he is bathed in perspiration. Then he inhales through both nostrils, making a noise like the male bee, and swallows the breath and suspends it, following kumbhaka with a slow expiration. This practice is preparatory to *rasananda yoga samadhi*.

Rasananda Yoga Samadhi

This practice is best done at midnight in absolute silence. Do bhramari kumbhaka and then slowly expel the breath, making a buzzing sound like that of a bee drunk with the nectar of the flower. This is produced by uttering the sound "ah" as low in the throat as possible, vibrating the palate, and continuing this practice until the tone can be made clear, when it will take on the characteristic sound of the bee drone. One focuses the mind on the center of this sound. The mind will become fixed and absorbed and one will experience intense joy. This practice will be effective only when kumbhaka can be done for several minutes.

Murchha Kumbhaka

The distinctive part of this practice is the use of the chin lock in exhalation. This practice renders the mind passive and quiet. Sit in siddhasana and inhale through both nostrils, producing the sound of rain. Swallow and do jalandhara and ashvini mudras. Then, with the pressure in the lower abdominal region, expel the air slowly, followed by an external kumbhaka, which will cause the mind to swoon, producing a sense of comfort. Should a trance occur, you can be certain kumbhaka is successful. To complete *murchha*, shakti chalana must be practiced with it.

Kevala Kumbhaka

In this practice the full length of the breath is confined in the body and nothing is exhaled. It is absolute suspension, performed without any physical or muscular effort. Through this practice sushumna becomes free of all impurities and the aim of pranayama is accomplished. This practice cures all diseases, promotes longevity, removes the darkness of ignorance for the aspirant, elevates the moral nature, purges all faults, and awakens shakti, thus achieving samadhi. The chitta can be directed anywhere and one will easily attain perfection in everything. One must already be skilled in the various pranayama practices and must be capable of perfect concentration of the mind, going as far as the level of absorption in which thoughts become visualized, before he undertakes *kevala kumbhaka*.

Traditionally, when the aspirant has perfected khechari

mudra (the retroversion of the tongue) and lives in the traditional subterranean retreat, he reduces his diet to that of rich milk, living on milk alone for six months. He then begins to live on ghee and milk for about a week, following which he abstains from all foods for a day or two. Then, consciously counting his respirations, he raises them to twice the normal number and practices this for some time. Then, filling the lungs with air, he shuts both nostrils, presses the epiglottis backward using the tip of the tongue, and swallows the tongue into the pharynx. He then suspends his breath, and at the same time focuses his gaze between the eyebrows or the tip of the nose. When his mind becomes quiet and absorbed, he attains spiritual power. When kumbhaka is completed, he should allow his mind to rest.

This may be performed three times a day, every three hours, or one may practice it five times a day: early morning, noon, twilight, midnight, and then in the fourth quarter of the night (4 a.m. to 8 a.m.). This absorbed state of breath suspension should be continued until success is obtained, and the practice should be gradually increased until one attains samadhi. Thus the aspirant produces a state of *manomani,* or fixedness of mind, at which point kevala should be practiced only once a day.

When the vayus are united and begin to move in sushumna the whole of the heart becomes open. The aspirant's body becomes glowingly healthy, and it emits a subtle sweet scent. His posture becomes firm. When yoga is thus perfected the aspirant masters the secrets of life and the universe, and it is said that the goddess of wisdom always dances on his tongue.

When the yogi can suspend his respiratory movements for 10 minutes 48 seconds, he can suspend the activity of the senses. Dharana, concentration, is attained when the breath can be held for 21 minutes 36 seconds; dhyana, meditation, when the breath is held for 43 minutes 12 seconds; and samadhi by holding the breath for 1 hour 26 minutes 24 seconds. When synthesized, these last three stages of yoga (concentration, meditation, and samadhi) are known as *samyama*.

When the yogi can perform kumbhaka for 2½ to 3 hours it is said that he will attain extraordinary powers, such as hearing sounds at great distances, seeing objects out of ordinary view, and covering long distances quickly. Many phenomena will occur that are generally considered impossible. However, if one ceases his meditative practices in order to pursue these powers, which are only a natural consequence in the process of his advancement, it means certain defeat for him and the end to further progress on the path. One may, however, exhibit his accomplishments for the purpose of encouraging other practicing aspirants.

The aspirant has mastery over all aspects of the earth when he can restrain his breath of life in the muladhara chakra with awareness for 2½ hours. He can conquer all forms of water when he can retain it in svadhishthana for 2½ hours, and he can conquer all forms of fire by being aware of his breath as it is retained in the manipura chakra. He can control air with his breath in the anahata for 2½ hours, and space when the breath is made stationary in vishuddha. In this way he obtains a knowledge and mastery of the five elements—these elements cannot limit him, for he enjoys them constantly and through these practices meets the universal life force.

When the yogi can restrain his breath for 3 hours he is able to unite his soul with the universal life force. At this state no worldly thoughts of any kind cross his mind, even momentarily. When one attains this state his passions become completely quieted, and he passes from the level of nature and the world to the divine and universal.

The yogis of ancient lore discovered that a human being is like a miniature universe, fully equipped with all possible means to attain enlightenment. When the aspirant determines to explore the potentials which lie dormant within himself he can attain the goal of life and serve others selflessly as well.

To practice the exercises on the path of the inner journey a disciplinary commitment is necessary. Aspirants who are on the path practice faithfully and attain peace, happiness, and bliss. Various are the methods for attaining this goal, but the yoga practices are precise and systematic in their essential nature. Self-discipline and regular practice are two main requisites. Those who are determined to walk on the path of light practice sincerely and regularly, and thus they finally attain the goal of life.

GLOSSARY

Abhyantara Internal kumbhaka: breath retention performed after the lungs are filled with air.

Adhama Pranayama The lowest stage of advanced pranayama, marked by profuse perspiration.

Adharakunda The place in the area of the muladhara chakra wherein kundalini sleeps.

Agni The fire element; one of the tattvas. Also referred to as tejas.

Agni Sara A yogic kriya which involves lifting the abdominal muscles and pulling up the pelvis gradually to strengthen the navel center. It is also known as the abdominal lift.

Ajna Chakra The sixth chakra, situated between the eyebrows; the seat of the mind.

Akasha The ether element; one of the tattvas.

Amavashya The new moon day. In the yogic tradition, the time when the sun and the moon meet at the muladhara chakra.

Amrita "Immortal." The nectar of immortality said to be produced when pranayama helps to dry semen; this force then ascends to return as nectar.

Anahata Chakra The heart center, the center of the air element; an important chakra for the practice of meditation.

Anahata Nada "Unstruck sound." The inner sound which can be heard through the practice of shambhava mudra or that sometimes emerges through mantra sadhana.

Annamaya Kosha The physical sheath; the physical body.

Apana One of the vayus; the vital force that has a tendency to move downward; the force which enables the functions of exhalation and excretion.

Apas The water element; one of the tattvas.

Asana Any of numerous yogic postures, some of which are necessary in the practice of pranayama.

Ashvini Mudra Contracting and releasing the anal muscle.

Ayurveda The ancient Indian medical science that promotes a long, healthy life.

Baddha Padmasana The bound lotus pose. A variation of the lotus pose in which one catches the toes with the hand of the same side from the back.

Bahya Kumbhaka External breath retention performed after completing an exhalation.

Bandha A lock, or control. There are many kinds of locks applied during the practice of pranayama; among them the root, navel, and chin locks are most important.

Basti A yogic method of enema for cleaning the colon.

Bhastrika A kind of pranayama involving forceful inhalation and exhalation, activating the lower abdominal muscles.

Bhedana To pierce or to penetrate, most often used in the sense of piercing the chakras and leading the kundalini to sahasrara.

Bhramari A kind of pranayama in which a sound like that of a humming bee is produced in the throat.

Bija Mantra Seed mantra. In the science of mantra certain letters or phonemes are supposed to be the foci of divine powers or vibratory patterns of certain elements.

Bindu A dot or point. In yogic tradition it represents seminal fluid or the point at the ajna chakra where ida and pingala terminate and the gateway to sahasrara begins.

Brahma Granthi The point between the eyebrows; the ajna chakra.

Brahma Nadi The central energy channel, also known as sushumna.

Brahmarandhra The location of sahasrara, the crown chakra, in the area of the soft spot at the crown of the head.

Buddhi The intellect, the decisive faculty.

Chakra A center of consciousness. Seven are most commonly known, representing seven states of consciousness.

Chhaya Purusha Sadhana The specific practice in which one gazes at one's shadow and develops the supernatural power of knowing future events.

Chitrini Nadi The nadi in the interior of sushumna through which kundalini completes its upward journey to sahasrara.

Chitta Mind-stuff; the storehouse of memory; the unconscious mind.

Devadatta Vayu A kind of vayu responsible for yawning.

Devata The divine force materialized in visual form.

Dhananjaya The vayu that is responsible for the ability to hiccough.

Dharana Concentration; the sixth rung of raja yoga.

Dhatu Dosha; one of the three fundamental constituents, or life essences, of the body: vata, pitta, kapha.

Dhauti A yogic technique for cleaning the throat passage and stomach by swallowing a long piece of wet cloth and then pulling it out.

Dhyana Meditation, the seventh rung of raja yoga.

Dosha Dhatu; one of the three vital principles of the body which regulate the metabolic and catabolic processes: vata, the air-like principle; pitta, the fire-like principle; and kapha, the substantial principle.

Foot Lock The position of the legs and feet as held in siddhasana.

Ganglion Impar The lowest ganglion of the sympathetic nervous system, located in front of the coccyx.

Ganglion of Ribes The uppermost ganglion of the sympathetic nervous system, located within the brain.

Ghee Clarified butter; an essential dietary ingredient during the practice of vigorous pranayamas.

Granthi Any of several points in the body where the finer forces reside in their latent form (e.g., the base of the spine, the navel center, the center between the eyebrows). Three main knots are known as rudra, vishnu, and brahma.

Guna "Quality." One of the three attributes of prakriti: sattva, rajas, tattva.

Ida One of the three nadis, corresponding to lunar energy and situated on the left side of the spinal column.

Jalandhara Bandha The chin lock, performed by placing the chin at the hollow of the throat in order to prevent the excessive energy produced through vigorous pranayama from moving toward the head.

Jiva The individual soul which identifies itself with the body-mind organism.

Kaki Mudra "Crow bill mudra." Drinking in the air through the mouth while the tongue is rolled lengthwise, making a shape similar to that of a crow, and exhaling through the nostrils. This has a cooling effect.

Kanda "Root." The area between the anus and the generative organ.

Kapalabhati A type of pranayama in which one exhales forcefully and inhales normally.

Kapha The heavy, substantial principle responsible for growth and metabolic processes. See also Dosha.

Karma Action. It includes the law of actions and reactions, the driving forces of one's present and future.

Kevala Kumbhaka A type of pranayama in which either the breath stops of its own accord, or a pause is created after many inhalations and exhalations and no effort is made to retain the breath.

Khechari Mudra Curling the tongue and tucking it in toward the palate.

Krikara The vayu which induces hunger and thirst as well as sneezing.

Kriya Any of various yogic purification practices.

Kumbhaka Suspension of breath; breath retention.

Kundalini Creative energy in a static state, the spiritual force itself, "the Grand Potential."

Kurma Vaya The force which governs involuntary expansion and contraction, such as the opening and closing of the eyelids.

Laya A specific path of yoga in which the mind is led to absorption in nada, the internal sound.

Lunar Breath Breathing predominantly through the left nostril.

Madhyama The intermediate stage of pranayama, in which one may feel a quivering sensation or a vibration throughout the body.

Maha Bandha A yogic lock performed by fixing the left heel underneath the perineum, and the right foot upon the left thigh. Then after inhaling fully, one locks the chin, holds the breath as long as possible, and exhales slowly. In the second round, the position of the heel and the foot is reversed.

Maha Mudra "Great mudra." Fixing the left heel underneath the perineum and holding the toes of the outstretched right foot.

Maha Vayu A supplementary vayu operating only on the physical plane that helps regulate the functioning of the brain.

Maha Vedha "Great penetration." An internal yogic kriya to force prana to enter the sushumna by leaving its usual course through ida and pingala.

Manas The faculty of thought experienced as a state of doubt and uncertainty.

Manduka Mudra "Frog mudra." Turning the tongue back, placing its tip on the soft palate, and then inhaling through the combined pressure of the tongue and soft palate.

Manipura "Filled with jewels." The third chakra, the center of fire, the navel center.

Manomani Fixedness of mind.

Manomaya Kosha The mental sheath. All the faculties of mind which veil the light of consciousness.

Mantra A set of syllables, sounds, or words, received from the teacher during initiation for meditation and spiritual advancement.

Mantra Yoga The path of yoga which emphasizes meditation on a mantra as the main means for enlightenment.

Matra The amount of time required to utter a short letter.

Matrika "Mother." Sanskrit letters and phonemes from which the mantras derive.

Maya The force through which the infinite is experienced as being finite, or the force because of which one mistakes the unreal for the real, and vice versa.

Medulla Oblongata The junction of the spinal cord and the brain.

Moksha The liberation which is attained upon realizing the true nature of the self. This is the state in which one is no longer subject to worldly influences.

Mudra A yogic gesture. There are various yogic mudras which, combined with asanas and bandhas (locks), are practiced as prerequisites for awakening kundalini.

Mula Bandha The root lock, performed by contracting the anal muscle upward.

Muladhara The root support chakra situated at the base of the spine, the center of the earth element.

Murchha Kumbhaka A special kind of breath retention performed with the intention to lead the mind into a trance state.

Nada The celestial sound that yogis hear internally. By contemplating on this sound the mind becomes focused and inward.

Nadi Energy channel. According to yoga manuals, there are 72,000 nadis, among which 14 are most important.

Nadi Shodhanam Channel purification, also known as alternate nostril breathing.

Naga One of the supplementary vayus, which performs the function of belching and also provides clarity of mind.

Nasagra Drishti The nasal gaze.

Nauli A cleansing kriya performed by rolling the abdominal muscles from one side to the other. This churning movement isolates the abdominal muscles, giving the impression of a continuous rolling movement through alternate contraction and relaxation.

Neti Nasal wash. The specific method of cleaning the nasal passage either with water or with a specially prepared soft string.

Ojas The finest of the primary constituents of the body. It is described as brilliance, human aura, vigor, or zeal.

Padmasana The lotus pose.

Patanjali Codifier of the science and practice of yoga. The author of the *Yoga Sutra*.

Pingala One of the three major energy channels, situated along the right side of the spinal column, corresponding to the solar energy in the body.

Pitta The fiery energy responsible for all the catabolic processes taking place in the body. See also Dosha.

Prakriti Matter; creative will. The creative force, possessed of three attributes: sattva, rajas, tamas. See also Purusha.

Prana Generally, the etheric life essence. Specifically, one of the five major vayus, marked by inhalation or the taking in of fresh life essence; the heart, lungs, and brain are considered to be the main seats of this vital force.

Pranamaya Kosha The energy sheath, which is subtler than the physical sheath and creates a bridge between the mental and physical sheaths.

Pranayama Expansion of or voluntary control over the pranic force.

Prithivi The earth element, the grossest tattva. Smell and solidity are its main qualities.

Puraka Inhalation. It is called puraka, "the filler," since one fills the lungs with air through inhalation. Later this air may be retained or expelled as required by the rules of pranayama.

Purusha Spirit; pure awareness. The witness of the force of prakriti.

Rahu The moon's north node. One of the nine planets which according to the ancient scientists of the East significantly affect the life force on earth, especially during the solar and lunar eclipses.

Rajas The force of activity and movement. One of the three attributes of prakriti.

Raja Yoga The royal path. The eightfold path as described by Patanjali in the *Yoga Sutra*.

Rasa The metabolized food essence.

Rasananda Yoga Samadhi Meditation on the sound induced through bhramari pranayama.

Rechaka Exhalation. It is called rechaka, "the releaser," since the air which has been taken in or retained is released through expiration.

Rudra Granthi The fiery knot which covers the two lowest chakras—muladhara and svadhishthana.

Sadhana Practice, spiritual endeavor.

Sadhanatita "Beyond practices." The regulation and control of wakefulness, dreaming, and deep sleep without relying on the cardiac temperatures at which the sensory organs ordinarily work. This is beyond the scope of sadhana since it can be done only by an accomplished yogi who remains in the state of turiya, in which empirical means and resources cannot be applied.

Sahasrara "Thousand-petaled." The crown chakra.

Sahita Kumbhaka A specific breath retention in which the mind is focused on some object besides, or in addition to, the breath.

Samadhi Spiritual absorption; the eighth rung of raja yoga.

Samana The pranic force which separates food nutrients from waste elements.

Samyama The continuum of concentration, meditation, and samadhi.

Sandhi "Juncture." The period when the breath is changing its predominance from one nostril to the other.

Sanskrit The language of the yogic scriptures. It is the most ancient language, possessing a rich literature on philosophy and spirituality.

Sarvangasana The shoulderstand.

Sattva The quality of light and illumination. One of the three attributes of prakriti.

Shakti "Power." The dynamic aspect of consciousness, the source of the manifest world and its activities. The polar opposite of shiva.

Shakti Chalana The awakening and moving of kundalini shakti.

Shakti Chalana Mudra Firmly holding the ankles with the hands while in vajrasana, thereby putting pressure on muladhara.

Shakti Nadi The sushumna, the innermost or central energy channel, through which the kundalini shakti travels.

Shambhava Mudra A yogic kriya in which one mentally focuses on the life force in the heart center, leaving the eyes open as if seeing everything.

Shiva Pure consciousness, existence, and bliss. In contrast to shakti, shiva is the static state of consciousness.

Siddhasana The accomplished pose, which is required exclusively in the practice of some of the advanced pranayamas.

Siddhi Any of numerous powers which are achieved through various yogic practices such as pranayama, mantra japa, etc.

Sitali Inhaling through the mouth and exhaling through the nostrils. This is quite similar to sitkari pranayama while applying manduka mudra.

Sitkari A way of inhaling through the mouth and exhaling through the nostrils that has a cooling effect on the body.

Solar Breath Breathing predominantly through the right nostril.

Sukhasana The easy pose. Sitting cross-legged with head, neck, and trunk straight.

Sukshma Dhyana Luminous concentration. Any of various visualization practices (e.g., chhaya purusha sadhana).

Superior Hypogastric Plexus A large collection of primarily sympathetic nerve bodies which send nerves to the pelvic organs.

Surya Bhedana Kumbhaka A specific type of breath retention in which one inhales through the right nostril to the fullest capacity and then, while applying the chin lock, retains the breath; then one exhales through the left nostril slowly and uninterruptedly.

Sushumna The wedding of day and night. The brahma nadi, also known as shakti nadi, the central channel through which kundalini travels and unites herself with shiva in sahasrara.

Svadhishthana "Her own abode." The second chakra.

Svara "Sound." The life force; prana.

Svara Yogi A yogi who advances on the spiritual path emphasizing the practice of svara, the life force.

Svarodaya "Rise of svara." The science which describes the subtleties of prana and the methods for expanding and controlling it.

Tamas The quality of sloth, inertia, heaviness, dullness. One of the three attributes of prakriti.

Tantra A branch of yoga which incorporates divergent disciplines such as hatha, kundalini, external rituals, meditation, and yantra.

Tattva Element. There are five gross elements: earth, water, fire, air, and ether.

Tejas Fire; one of the five tattvas; also referred to as agni. It sometimes represents the catabolic force, the force through which the digestive process takes place.

Trataka Gazing at an external object; a practice designed to enhance one-pointedness.

Tripatha Sthana The point where ida, pingala, and sushumna meet; the ajna chakra.

Turiya The fourth, transcendental, state of consciousness, beyond the states of waking, dreaming, and deep sleep.

Udana The vital force through which upward movement takes place and also that which forces air out of the lungs.

Uddiyana Bandha Navel lock performed by lifting the abdominal muscles and pushing them toward the rib cage, thus creating a cavity in the stomach and navel area.

Ujjayi A type of pranayama performed by inhaling through both nostrils, expanding the chest, and making a sobbing sound by closing the glottis at the completion of the inhalation. The breath is retained in the chin lock position and then air is exhaled through either the left nostril or both nostrils; the glottis remains partially closed, producing a sound of a low uniform pitch.

Unmani A state beyond the mind: the state of mind in which no objects or thought constructs exist.

Unmani Mudra Contemplation upon the void.

Urdhva Retas Upward traveling. A practice whereby—using pranayamas, locks, and mudras—one forces the seminal fluid to move upward and does not allow it to be dissipated.

Uttama The highest stage of pranayama, in which the practitioner feels that the body is being suspended in the air.

Vajrasana The thunderbolt pose; also known as the pelvic pose or the adamantine pose.

Vata Vayu, the vital force. One of the major life essences. See also Dosha.

Vayu Vata; literally, the air element; that which flows. At a more subtle level it is not merely air but the medium in which air exists and the force which holds all aspects of life together.

Vayu Siddhi Perfection over vayu—the ability to leave the ground and rise in the air while seated in padmasana.

Vena Cava The largest vein in the body. It returns blood to the heart.

Vishnu Granthi The second granthi, the knot at the manipura chakra.

Vishuddha Chakra The throat center, the fifth chakra. The center of space.

Vritti A mode or modification of mind; a thought construct.

Vyana The vital force which helps supply blood and energy to the senses and which travels throughout the body.

Yoni Mudra A yogic method for cleaning the bladder, as well as a method for forcing the sexual energy to travel upward; also known as vajroli mudra.

About Swami Rama

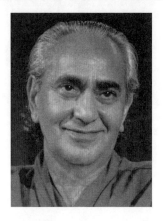

ONE OF THE greatest adepts, teachers, writers, and humanitarians of the 20th century, Swami Rama is the founder of the Himalayan Institute. Born in the Himalayas, he was raised from early childhood by the great Himalayan sage, Bengali Baba. Under the guidance of his master he traveled from monastery to monastery and studied with a variety of Himalayan saints and sages, including his grandmaster, who was living in a remote region of Tibet. In addition to this intense spiritual training, Swami Rama received higher education in both India and Europe. From 1949 to 1952, he held the prestigious position of Shankaracharya of Karvirpitham in South India. Thereafter, he returned to his master to receive further training at his cave monastery, and finally, in 1969, came to the United States, where he founded the Himalayan Institute. His best-known work, *Living with the Himalayan Masters*, reveals the many facets of this singular adept and demonstrates his embodiment of the living Himalayan Tradition.

HIMALAYAN INSTITUTE®

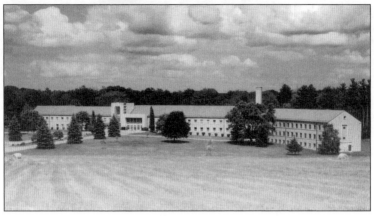

The main building of the Himalayan Institute headquarters near Honesdale, Pennsylvania

The Himalayan Institute

A leader in the field of yoga, meditation, spirituality, and holistic health, the Himalayan Institute is a nonprofit international organization dedicated to serving humanity through educational, spiritual, and humanitarian programs. The mission of the Himalayan Institute is to inspire, educate, and empower all those who seek to experience their full potential.

Founded in 1971 by Swami Rama of the Himalayas, the Himalayan Institute and its varied activities and programs exemplify the spiritual heritage of mankind that unites East and West, spirituality and science, ancient wisdom and modern technology.

Our international headquarters is located on a beautiful 400-acre campus in the rolling hills of the Pocono Mountains of northeastern Pennsylvania. Our spiritually vibrant community and peaceful setting provide the perfect atmosphere for seminars and retreats, residential programs, and holistic health services. Students from all over the world join us to attend diverse programs on subjects such as hatha yoga, meditation, stress reduction, ayurveda, and yoga and tantra philosophy.

In addition, the Himalayan Institute draws on roots in the yoga tradition to serve our members and community through the following programs, services, and products:

Mission Programs

The essence of the Himalayan Institute's teaching mission flows from the timeless message of the Himalayan Masters, and is echoed in our on-site mission programming. Their message is to first become aware of the reality within ourselves, and then to build a bridge between our inner and outer worlds.

Our mission programs express a rich body of experiential wisdom and are offered year-round. They include seminars, retreats, and professional certifications that bring you the best of an authentic yoga tradition, addressed to a modern audience. Join us on campus for our Mission Programs to find wisdom from the heart of the yoga tradition, guidance for authentic practice, and food for your soul.

Wisdom Library and Mission Membership

The Himalayan Institute online Wisdom Library curates the essential teachings of the living Himalayan Tradition. This offering is a unique counterpart to our in-person Mission Programs, empowering students by providing online learning resources to enrich their study and practice outside the classroom.

Our Wisdom Library features multimedia blog content, livestreams, podcasts, downloadable practice resources, digital courses, and an interactive Seeker's Forum. These teachings capture our Mission Faculty's decades of study, practice, and teaching experience, featuring new content as well as the timeless teachings of Swami Rama and Pandit Rajmani Tigunait.

We invite seekers and students of the Himalayan Tradition to become a Himalayan Institute Mission Member, which grants unlimited access to the Wisdom Library. Mission Membership offers a way for you to support our shared commitment to service, while deepening your study and practice in the living Himalayan Tradition.

Spiritual Excursions

Since 1972, the Himalayan Institute has been organizing pilgrimages for spiritual seekers from around the world. Our spiritual excursions follow the traditional pilgrimage routes where adepts of the Himalayas lived and practiced. For thousands of years, pilgrimage has been an essential part of yoga sadhana, offering spiritual seekers the opportunity to experience the transformative power of living shrines of the Himalayan Tradition.

Global Humanitarian Projects

The Himalayan Institute's humanitarian mission is yoga in action—offering spiritually grounded healing and transformation to the world. Our humanitarian projects serve impoverished communities in India, Mexico, and Cameroon through rural empowerment and environmental regeneration. By putting yoga philosophy into practice, our programs are empowering communities globally with the knowledge and tools needed for a lasting social transformation at the grassroots level.

Publications

The Himalayan Institute publishes over 60 titles on yoga, philosophy, spirituality, science, ayurveda, and holistic health. These include the best-selling books *Living with the Himalayan Masters* and *The Science of Breath*, by Swami Rama; *The Power of Mantra and the Mystery of Initiation, From Death to Birth, Tantra Unveiled,* and two commentaries on the *Yoga Sutra—The Secret of the Yoga Sutra: Samadhi Pada* and *The Practice of the Yoga Sutra: Sadhana Pada*— by Pandit Rajmani Tigunait, PhD; and the award-winning *Yoga: Mastering the Basics* by Sandra Anderson and Rolf Sovik, PsyD. These books are for everyone: the interested reader, the spiritual novice, and the experienced practitioner.

PureRejuv Wellness Center

For over 40 years, the PureRejuv Wellness Center has fulfilled part of the Institute's mission to promote healthy and sustainable lifestyles. PureRejuv combines Eastern philosophy and Western medicine in an integrated approach to holistic health—nurturing balance and healing at home and at work. We offer the opportunity to find healing and renewal through on-site wellness retreats and individual wellness services, including therapeutic massage and bodywork, yoga therapy, ayurveda, biofeedback, natural medicine, and one-on-one consultations with our integrative medical staff.

Total Health Products

The Himalayan Institute, the developer of the original Neti Pot, manufactures a health line specializing in traditional and modern ayurvedic supplements and body care. We are dedicated to holistic and natural living by providing products using non-GMO components, petroleum-free biodegrading plastics, and eco-friendly packaging that has the least impact on the environment. Part of every purchase supports our Global Humanitarian projects, further developing and reinforcing our core mission of spirituality in action.

For further information about our programs, humanitarian projects, and products:

call: 800.822.4547
e-mail: info@HimalayanInstitute.org
write: The Himalayan Institute
         952 Bethany Turnpike
         Honesdale, PA 18431
or visit: HimalayanInstitute.org

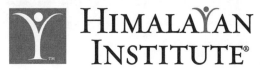
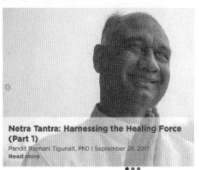

LIVING WITH THE HIMALAYAN MASTERS

SWAMI RAMA

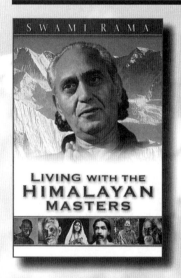

In this classic spiritual autobiography, hear the message of
Sri Swami Rama, one of the greatest sages of the 20th century.
As he shares precious experiences with his beloved master,
Sri Bengali Baba, and many other well-known and hidden
spiritual luminaries, you will have a glimpse of the living
tradition of the Himalayan Masters.

This spiritual treasure records Swami Rama's personal quest
for enlightenment and gives profound insights into the living
wisdom that is the core of his spiritual mission and legacy.
This living wisdom continues to enlighten seekers even
today, long after Swamiji's maha-samadhi in 1996, sharing
the timeless blessing of the sages of the Himalayan Tradition.

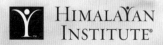

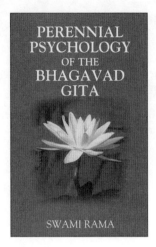

Perennial Psychology of the Bhagavad Gita
Swami Rama

With the guidance and commentary of Himalayan Master Swami Rama, you can explore the wisdom of the Bhagavad Gita, which allows one to be vibrant and creative in the external world while maintaining a state of inner tranquility. This commentary on the Bhagavad Gita is a unique opportunity to see the Gita through the perspective of a master yogi, and is an excellent version for practitioners of yoga meditation. Spiritual seekers, psychotherapists, and students of Eastern studies will all find a storehouse of wisdom in this volume.

Paperback, 6" x 9", 479 pages
$19.95, ISBN 978-0-89389-090-2

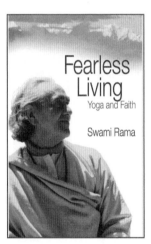

Fearless Living: Yoga and Faith
Swami Rama

Learn to live without fear—to trust a higher power, a divine purpose. In this collection of anecdotes from the astonishing life of Swami Rama, you will understand that there is a way to move beyond mere faith and into the realm of personal revelation. Through his astonishing life experiences we learn about ego and humility, see how to overcome fears that inhibit us, discover sacred places and rituals, and learn the importance of a one-pointed, positive mind. Swami Rama teaches us to see with the eyes of faith and move beyond our self-imposed limitations.

Paperback with flaps, 6" x 9", 160 pages
$12.95, ISBN 978-0-89389-251-7

To order: 800-822-4547
Email: mailorder@HimalayanInstitute.org
Visit: HimalayanInstitute.org

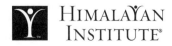

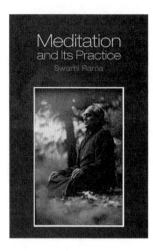

Meditation and Its Practice
Swami Rama

In this practical guide to inner life, Swami Rama teaches us how to slip away from the mental turbulence of our ordinary thought processes into an infinite reservoir of consciousness. This clear, concise meditation manual provides systematic guidance in the techniques of meditation - a powerful tool for transforming our lives and increasing our experience of peace, joy, creativity, and inner tranquility.

Paperback, 6" x 9", 128 pages
$12.95, ISBN 978-0-89389-153-4

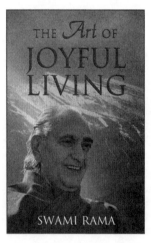

The Art of Joyful Living
Swami Rama

In *The Art of Joyful Living*, Swami Rama imparts a message of inspiration and optimism: that you are responsible for making your life happy and emanating that happiness to others. This book shows you how to maintain a joyful view of life even in difficult times.

It contains sections on transforming habit patterns, working with negative emotions, developing strength and willpower, developing intuition, spirituality in loving relationships, learning to be your own therapist, understanding the process of meditation, and more!

Paperback, 6" x 9", 198 pages
$15.95, ISBN 978-0-89389-236-4

To order: 800-822-4547
Email: mailorder@HimalayanInstitute.org
Visit: HimalayanInstitute.org

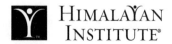

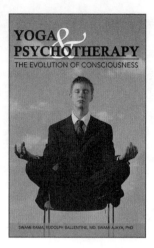

Yoga and Psychotherapy
The Evolution of Consciousness
Swami Rama, Rudolph Ballentine, MD,
Swami Ajaya, PhD

For thousands of years yoga has offered what Western therapists are currently seeking: a way to achieve the total health of body, mind, emotions, and spirit. *Yoga and Psychotherapy* provides a unique comparison of modern therapy and traditional methods. Drawing upon a rich diversity of experience, the authors give us detailed examples of how the ancient findings of yoga can be used to supplement or replace some of the less complete Western theories and techniques.

Paperback, 6"x 9", 305 pages
$15.95, ISBN 978-0-89389-036-0

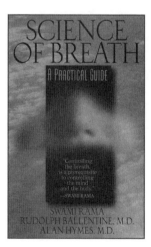

Science of Breath
A Practical Guide
Swami Rama, Rudolph Ballentine, MD,
Alan Hymes, MD

Proper breathing helps us achieve physical and mental health and attain higher states of consciousness. *Science of Breath* shows us how. It describes the anatomy and physiology of breathing, as well as the subtle yogic science of prana. Basic yogic breathing techniques are explained so that we can immediately begin working with this powerful science.

Paperback, 6"x 9", 119 pages
$12.95, ISBN 978-0-89389-151-0

To order: 800-822-4547
Email: mailorder@HimalayanInstitute.org
Visit: HimalayanInstitute.org

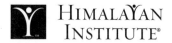

HIMALAYAN
INSTITUTE®

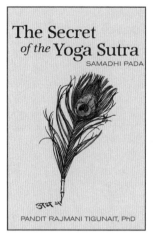

The Secret of the Yoga Sutra
Samadhi Pada
Pandit Rajmani Tigunait, PhD

The Yoga Sutra is the living source wisdom of the yoga tradition, and is as relevant today as it was 2,200 years ago when it was codified by the sage Patanjali. Using this ancient yogic text as a guide, we can unlock the hidden power of yoga, and experience the promise of yoga in our lives. By applying its living wisdom in our practice, we can achieve the purpose of life: lasting fulfillment and ultimate freedom.

Paperback, 6" x 9", 331 pages
$24.95, ISBN 978-0-89389-277-7

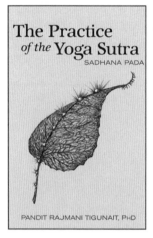

The Practice of the Yoga Sutra
Sadhana Pada
Pandit Rajmani Tigunait, PhD

In Pandit Tigunait's practitioner-oriented commentary series, we see this ancient text through the filter of scholarly understanding and experiential knowledge gained through decades of advanced yogic practices. Through *The Secret of the Yoga Sutra* and *The Practice of the Yoga Sutra*, we receive the gift of living wisdom he received from the masters of the Himalayan Tradition, leading us to lasting happiness.

Paperback, 6" x 9", 389 Pages
$24.95, ISBN 978-0-89389-279-1

To order: 800-822-4547
Email: mailorder@HimalayanInstitute.org
Visit: HimalayanInstitute.org

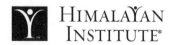

HIMALAYAN
INSTITUTE®

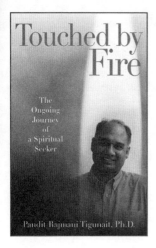

Touched by Fire
Pandit Rajmani Tigunait, PhD

This vivid autobiography of a remarkable spiritual leader—
Pandit Rajmani Tigunait, PhD—reveals his experiences and
encounters with numerous teachers, sages, and his master, the
late Swami Rama of the Himalayas. His well-told journey is
filled with years of disciplined study and the struggle to master
the lessons and skills passed to him. *Touched by Fire* brings
Western culture a glimpse of Eastern philosophies in a clear,
understandable fashion, and provides numerous photographs
showing a part of the world many will never see for themselves.

Paperback with flaps, 6" x 9", 296 pages
$16.95, ISBN 978-0-89389-239-5

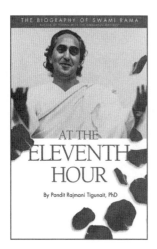

At the Eleventh Hour
Pandit Rajmani Tigunait, PhD

This book is more than the biography of a great sage—it is a
revelation of the many astonishing accomplishments Swami
Rama achieved in his life. These pages serve as a guide to the
more esoteric and advanced practices of yoga and tantra not
commonly taught or understood in the West. And they bring
you to holy places in India, revealing why these sacred sites are
important and how to go about visiting them. The wisdom in
these stories penetrates beyond the power of words.

Paperback with flaps, 6" x 9", 448 pages
$18.95, ISBN 978-0-89389-211-1

To order: 800-822-4547
Email: mailorder@HimalayanInstitute.org
Visit: HimalayanInstitute.org

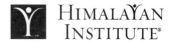

HIMALAYAN
INSTITUTE®

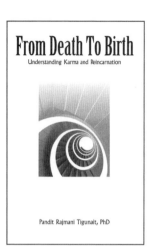

Pandit Rajmani Tigunait, PhD

From Death to Birth
Pandit Rajmani Tigunait, PhD

From Death to Birth takes us along the soul's journey from death to birth, dispelling the frequent misconceptions about this subject by revealing little-known but powerful truths. Through a series of lively stories drawn from the ancient scriptures and his own experience, Pandit Tigunait reveals what karma really is, how we can create it, why it becomes our destiny, and how we can use it to shape the future of our dreams.

Paperback, 6" x 9", 216 pages
$15.95, ISBN 978-0-89389-147-3

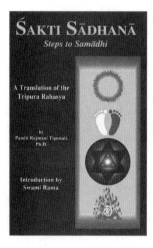

Sakti Sadhana
Pandit Rajmani Tigunait, PhD

The knowledge that enlightens the aspiring student into the mystery of life here and hereafter is the *Tripura Rahasya*. This text is one of the most significant scriptures in the tradition of tantra yoga. Its beauty lies in the fact that it expounds the lofty knowledge of inner truth while systematically offering practical instructions on *sakti sadhana*—the task of awakening the dormant fire within and leading it to higher awareness, or the highest chakra.

Paperback, 6" x 9", 196 pages
$10.95, ISBN 978-0-89389-140-4

To order: 800-822-4547
Email: mailorder@HimalayanInstitute.org
Visit: HimalayanInstitute.org

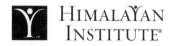

HIMALAYAN INSTITUTE®

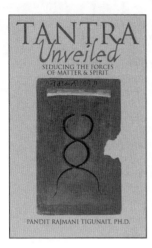

Tantra Unveiled
Pandit Rajmani Tigunait, PhD

This powerful book describes authentic tantra, what
distinguishes it from other spiritual paths, and how the
tantric way combines hatha yoga, meditation, visualization, ayurveda, and other disciplines. Taking us back to
ancient times, Pandit Tigunait shares his experiences
with tantric masters and the techniques they taught him.
Tantra Unveiled is most valuable for those who wish to
live the essence of tantra—practicing spirituality while
experiencing a rich outer life.

Paperback, 6" x 9", 152 pages
$14.95, ISBN 978-0-89389-158-9

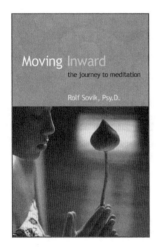

Moving Inward
Rolf Sovik, PsyD

Rolf Sovik shows readers of all levels how to transition
from asanas to meditation. Combining practical advice on
breathing and relaxation with timeless asana postures, he
systematically guides us through the process. This book
provides a five-stage plan to basic meditation, step-by-
step guidelines for perfect postures, and six methods for
training the breath. Both the novice and the advanced
student will benefit from Sovik's startling insights into the
mystery of meditation.

Paperback, 6" x 9", 197 pages
$14.95, ISBN 978-0-89389-247-0

To order: 800-822-4547
Email: mailorder@HimalayanInstitute.org
Visit: HimalayanInstitute.org

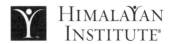

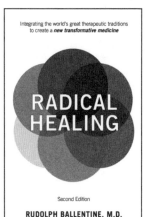

Radical Healing
Integrating the World's Greatest Therapeutic Traditions To Create a New Transformative Medicine
Rudolph Ballentine, MD

This second edition of *Radical Healing*—revised, expanded, and updated—presents a new vision of health care, one that integrates the holistic traditions of Ayurveda, homeopathy, Traditional Chinese Medicine, and other herbal medicinal traditions. It shows how they overlap, differ, and can be combined for dynamic healing and personal transformation. Includes a Self-Help guide to natural remedies and teatments for over 100 common ailments.

Paperback, 6"x 9", 644 pages
$19.95, ISBN 978-0-89389-308-8

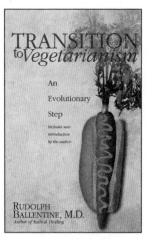

Transition to Vegetarianism
An Evolutionary Step
Rudolph Ballentine, MD

Written by the author of the popular classics *Diet and Nutrition* and *Radical Healing*, this book explores the health issues surrounding vegetarianism and helps the aspiring vegetarian make the transition in a way that provides the greatest health benefits. *Transition to Vegetarianism* is well researched, easy to ready, and an excellent resource for both the seasoned and would-be vegetarian.

Paperback, 6"x 9", 300 pages
$16.95, ISBN 978-0-89389-104-6

To order: 800-822-4547
Email: mailorder@HimalayanInstitute.org
Visit: HimalayanInstitute.org

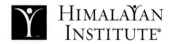